DARE TO THRIVE

How to Overcome Chronic Health Issues and Live Life Well

VICKI ROBINSON

First published by Ultimate World Publishing 2022
Copyright © 2022 Vicki Robinson

ISBN

Paperback: 978-1-922714-52-7
Ebook: 978-1-922714-53-4

Cover design: Ultimate World Publishing
Layout and typesetting: Ultimate World Publishing
Editor: Emily Riches
Cover photo license: Bess Hamitii-Shutterstock.com

Ultimate World Publishing
Diamond Creek,
Victoria Australia 3089
www.writeabook.com.au

ULTIMATE WORLD
—— PUBLISHING ——

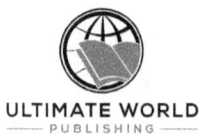

Note from the Author

The information in this book is not intended to replace a one on one relationship with a qualified health care professional, and is not intended as medical advice. It is the sharing of knowledge and information from the research and experience of Vicki Robinson.

Warning: some of the material may be sensitive to the reader. The topics covered include serious illness and death, including suicide.

If you find the content distressing, please reach out to www.lifeline. org.au or consult your medical provider.

Contents

Introduction

I have worked in health and fitness for most of my adult life as a registered nurse, personal trainer, and holistic health and wellness coach. Even when not working, it has always been my passion to learn as much as I can about our wonderful human bodies.

Science had always been my favourite subject at school and human biology topped it off. I had witnessed my patients' and clients' struggles. I knew that my lifestyle wasn't always perfect but none of it prepared me for the shock of receiving my own diagnosis of multiple sclerosis.

On my youngest child's 12th birthday, I was heading to the local hospital for my first infusion. I just had time to buy a cake before my appointment. It should have been easy but my legs would not cooperate. I made it home with the cake but had to call a friend to take me to the hospital. It was a long walk and she had to grab a wheelchair as I just couldn't make it under my own steam.

My neurologist had told me that infusions would make me feel much better. However, as treatment continued, I felt worse and worse. If I'm honest with myself, I became more and more depressed with constant thoughts that my life was over. I would have put an end to my misery if I was able but I couldn't even manage to get down the stairs or drive my car.

That was until I made a decision. I had been trained in the traditional medical model as a registered nurse where we were taught each body system individually. It was only through my own experience that I learned the importance of viewing the body holistically. All parts work together in a synchronistic way to create the amazing vessel that we call our body.

It is capable of reversing damage, healing… when we remove what is harmful and give it what it needs.

Friends have long urged me to write my story. I have often agreed that, yes, maybe I should. It was the pandemic that prompted me to finally take up the challenge. As events unfolded globally, more and more it was chronic health conditions that stood out as risk factors for adverse outcomes.

I knew that it was possible to improve health in a number of ways. I decided it was time. In the first four chapters, I will take you on a journey through parts of my story. Not everything in micro detail. Just enough for context. My hope is that it will ignite a spark or 'aha!' moment that readers can relate to.

I have also shared some stories about my clients and patients as examples to aid in further understanding.

The remainder of the book is a crash course on our biology and some of the ways it can go wrong. More importantly, my aim is to focus on putting things right. It is the product of my combined learning, training and experience. It's a big task! There is vastly more on each individual subject than could fit in a single book. My intention is to explain key points with enough detail to set you on your own path to healing.

We all have a different experience of even the same event. We are all individuals with individual circumstances. Not everyone will identify with everything. My list is by no means complete. It is ordered in the way that I approach my clients.

My aim is to give hope and awareness. When we are open to possibility, big changes can – and do – happen. I make no assertions as to any particular outcome. We are all on our own journey. What could be possible for you? The one thing that I can say with unshakeable certainty is that, 'if nothing changes, nothing changes.' Read on, and let's see.

PART ONE

CHAPTER ONE

We Live What We Learn

———————•———————

'*Parents are the ultimate role models for children. Every word, movement and action has an effect. No other person or outside force has a greater influence on a child than the parent.*'
– Bob Keeshan

Growing up, and throughout most of my adult life, I thought my life was fairly normal. I didn't really understand how relevant childhood experiences are on your health as you grow up. Knowing what I know now that was not necessarily true: my life was eventful and hardly normal.

I was conceived out of wedlock and my parents were both quite young. My mother was 18, my father 20, so they were not even legal adults as it remained age 21 until 1974. It really was not the done thing back in the day, so I imagine that they felt a degree of shame as it would have been a major inconvenience for their families. I was born around five months after they married so no doubt it was a rush and not exactly the fairy tale that young girls hope for. On top of that, with help from their parents, they bought their first home. My mother used to like telling me that she had painted the ceiling with a two-inch paint brush while very pregnant with me.

It is now known that early bonding between a mother and the child is vitally important for the child's development and wellbeing. And it's fair to say that I wasn't born into an easy time for my parents. My father was just out of university and starting his career as an electronics engineer. His parents, I would later find out, did not believe that I was his child. They were of the view that my mother had tricked him into marriage by claiming that he was the father. His father passed away when I was three years old from lung cancer.

My mother's mother was quite unwell. She had suffered with anxiety and depression for most of her adult life. She had divorced my grandfather, as he was violent, when my mother was two years old. My mother had a prominent birthmark on her neck. When she was reunited with her father many years later, he said, 'I'm sorry, I think I did that.' My grandmother was in and out of psychiatric hospitals her entire life. By my mother's account, I learned to walk on the lawns of the psychiatric hospital.

So, it's quite possible that my mother wasn't always fully present for me. She said that I was a very independent child, even making my own bed by the age of two. I find that hard to imagine, but maybe that was the case. Throughout my life, I have always tried to maintain my independence. It is one of my highest values.

My father was moving quite quickly with his career. Around the time my sister was born, when I was three years old, we moved to Woomera. It was just a little village out in the middle of the desert in South Australia: a restricted area containing housing for military and civilian staff at a nearby rocket launching facility. I remember the military-style checkpoints at the entry to the town.

There was only one shop: a milk bar that was open one day a week. Mum had to drive a short distance to Pimba to 'shop.' It was a small town but really not much more than a railway siding. There, the tea and sugar train would arrive once a week. All shopping was done on the train, and it even had a hairdresser and library. There was no platform. We had to climb what seemed like a very big ladder.

I started school there and have a lot of good memories, like getting into trouble for playing in the mud. We were in the desert and rain was a big deal. Some of my classmates had never experienced it before. We collected tadpoles that turned into frogs in two days. Besides, not too many kids actually got to witness rockets being fired from their front porch, or walk on a salt lake.

By the time I was six, we moved to the lower Blue Mountains and my second sister was born. My mother was also fostering a second baby whose mother had postnatal depression. I remember standing on a chair to hang nappies on the line. With two newborns and two young girls, I imagine it was a very busy household.

Later that year, we had devastating bushfires. I remember being at school and seeing the scary red and black sky. Fires came in so quickly on three fronts that it wasn't possible to evacuate. My father had to run a roadblock to get home. I remember him describing the fire leaping the road behind him. We had to just sit tight and wait it out.

My mother had been told to fill up anything she could with water before the water mains were turned off. I remember we waited it out on our front patio in a wading pool filled with water. As we sat there, we watched the flames leap through the trees and over the top of the house. Luckily our house was spared, but seven houses around us were lost. To this day, I have a really uneasy feeling whenever I smell smoke or see that colour in the sky.

It is now believed that early traumatic experiences are stored within the nervous system of the body. They're also stored within the subconscious mind as a means to keep us safe in later life. It's possible that some of my early experiences were partly responsible for my experiences and choices in later life.

Life goes on however and my father's career was progressing. Around my eighth birthday, we moved to Canberra. We lived in a hotel for a while before we moved into a rented house. I started at a new school where I didn't really fit in. It was late in the year and I remember being given the humiliating part of a flower in the school pantomime. Of course, I knew it was too late for them to accommodate me, so I was included but felt left out at the same time. On top of that, because we weren't intending to be there for a long time, I didn't even have the uniform. I was the odd kid out and I remember being teased and picked on. The other kids even laughed at me for the content of my sandwiches.

Eventually my parents built our new home and I again started in a new school. This time it was a brand-new school just starting out in a new area in Canberra, which meant that everybody was new and out of uniform. I remember spending time helping my father in the garden, watching him as he worked on the family car or laughing as he danced around wearing a dress that my mother made for herself so that she could pin the hem.

I was ten when my mother was in hospital. She was expecting my third sister and there were complications. She had been expecting twins but lost one. Looking back, it seemed like she was in hospital for a very long time. Likely longer for my father who somehow looked after the three of us while still working. I remember lots of visits to the hospital and to the cafeteria for ice cream.

My third sister was born prematurely. She was a really unwell baby. I remember my father giving her physiotherapy. She had lung problems and needed some help to clear them. I learned to help a lot around the house. Not long after she was born, we moved to another new house. We still attended the same primary school, which was fine.

But then, I remember one Christmas morning when I was 12 years old. My grandparents had come to stay for Christmas. My grandmother came up from the garage, which was underneath our house. My grandfather asked her what she had been doing. She replied, 'Nothing, I've just been down in the shed.' That's what she called the garage. He smelled her breath and asked, 'What have you done?'

My father went straight down the stairs and came back up with a bottle of paint thinner. It was half empty. Then things happened pretty quickly. My father swept my grandmother up and carried her down to the car with my grandfather. My mother apparently phoned a friend and asked her to pick the four of us up. Leaving the four of us behind, they all raced off to the hospital.

The rest of that day, I don't recall much at all. I don't think we had Christmas that year. For the next six months, life was visits to the hospital and the psychiatric ward where my grandmother was. My grandfather had returned to Adelaide as he had to work. So, my mother was carting us all in and out of the hospital visiting my grandmother. She had an old car that had to be push-started and that was my job. As long as she parked on a slight slope, I could manage it.

I didn't understand it at the time but my grandmother received multiple rounds of electroconvulsive shock therapy. She apparently was never quite the same again. Remarkably, she completely recovered from the chemical burns in her throat and oesophagus. She would be in and out of care for the rest of her life. A sleep study many years later showed that she was unable to achieve proper sleep.

Eventually, my grandmother was released from the hospital. My grandfather came and they returned back home to Adelaide. Life settled into some sort of normal. Mum had returned to work for a while but had a car accident. She had quite a serious whiplash injury that was going to require surgery. My parents had only recently returned from a visit to the surgeon in Melbourne. She was booked in for surgery in a few months.

By then I was in high school, 14 years old, and one morning I got the call to come to the principal's office. Normally a call to come to the office meant that you were in really big trouble. So, I went with a sense of trepidation, thinking, 'Oh no, what have I done?' Only to be told, 'Your next-door neighbour is coming to pick you up. There's been a problem at home.' I then started thinking, 'Okay, a problem at home, phew, I'm not in trouble.'

Our next-door neighbour came to pick me up. I don't even remember her name. I asked her what had happened. She said, 'I can't tell you,

you'll find out when we get you home.' As we drove up the street, I could see my father's car in the driveway. He had dropped me off at school in the morning on his way to work as usual. He would have then dropped my youngest sister at her babysitter, before taking my other two sisters to their primary school.

So, my immediate thoughts went to my mother. What had happened to her? But as I got to the front door, I was greeted by my mother who told me, 'Your father's dead.' In my mind, I thought, 'No, that couldn't possibly be true. How could it be true? His car was in the driveway.'

I said, 'No, you're lying where is he?' My poor mother! I can't imagine what that must have been like. She was 33 years old with four children 14 and under – the youngest, only three. She had just lost her husband out of the blue. Life became very different.

My father's death was so sudden that there was a coroner's inquest, which meant that we couldn't have a funeral; we could only have a memorial service. They had discovered a drug, digoxin, in his system that shouldn't have been there. It would not, or should not, have been given by the ambulance or at the hospital in the emergency room.

He had just finished a course of antibiotics the day before as he had tonsillitis. The bottle had gone out with the garbage collection on the morning he died. My mother wondered if he had been given the wrong medication. He had been prescribed a capsule but had been taking a tablet. I remember a visit to our family GP where he showed my mother that the antibiotic tablet and the digoxin tablet were almost impossible to tell apart. The chemist's records were checked by the coroner but were inconclusive.

Then some of my father's relatives started accusing my mother of having something to do with my father's death. We then had detectives with a search warrant searching the house, looking for evidence. Digoxin is actually a derivative of digitalis, a plant commonly known as foxglove. I remember being sent out, gardening book in hand, with two big burly detectives. I had to show them that we definitely did not have any digitalis growing in our garden. I remember they searched through my mother's belongings as well. It must have been very traumatic for her.

My mother had surgery scheduled that had to go ahead. She needed a bone graft to stabilise her neck. She went into survival mode. She had to get through the surgery alone and also look after her children. We were farmed out amongst friends while she went to Melbourne. I stayed with the neighbours as someone had to feed the cats and my sister's guinea pig. Some friends drove me to Melbourne to visit mum in the hospital. There I met a nurse who would set the course of my life.

Mum had to be flown home lying flat. She had to pay for seven seats on the flight to accommodate the stretcher and have a nurse escort. The nurse was the same one I met in the hospital. She stayed with us for a couple of days and I spent a lot of time talking with her. For a long time, I had wanted to be a vet. That was until I accompanied an elderly neighbour to the vet. I often fed her cat and he was to be put down. Watching the procedure, I decided I couldn't possibly kill an animal. I don't remember everything that we talked about, but by the time she left I was determined to become a nurse.

We then had a live-in nanny, as mum had a long recovery ahead of her. Sally was a young girl, about 19 years old, who treated us like she was in charge of a military operation. It was a disaster. If we were not out of bed by seven o'clock in the morning, fully dressed with our beds made we didn't get breakfast. Very tough. Not exactly what a family with traumatised kids needed. We hadn't even buried our father yet. I don't remember exactly how long it was before I begged my mother to send Sally away.

We had some help with shopping and meal preparation for a while, but I think money ran out. Then I had to step up and take on a lot of extra responsibility. Eventually, life got back to somewhat normal. My mother's surgery had been successful. We were finally able to say goodbye to my father perhaps six months after his passing.

The coroner had not given my mother any comfort. On my father's death certificate were the words: 'How and by what means he came to his death I am unable to ascertain.' We returned home from the funeral to find a jar of honey at the doorstep with a note that read, 'For when sore throats are better.' It was from one of my father's particularly nasty relatives.

I was around 15 when I travelled with my sisters on an overnight bus to Adelaide to stay with my mother's parents. My father's mother also lived in Adelaide and she would often take us on outings. I remember one day she had taken us to the beach. I was sitting in the car with her while we watched my sisters play. She told me that she didn't think that I was my father's child. My mother had apparently tricked him into believing he was my father. She had to accept me anyway. Grief does strange things. I never saw my grandmother cry, not even at her son's funeral.

I remember being very upset, so much so that my mother found the money to fly us all home. I vowed to never speak to my grandmother again. Her comments had really hurt. Somehow, my mother managed to repair the relationship between us. Encyclopaedia Britannica to the rescue! There was a distant relative famous enough to have an entry. I remember mum insisting that my father had the same shaped nose, as did I. It worked, and my grandmother and I became close again.

By the time I was 17, mum had started a new career as a real estate agent. She decided that it was time to move house. The house she chose was being sold because of a divorce settlement. She started going out with one of the previous owners. They married not long after I turned 18. Shortly after, I left home, moving to Sydney to start my nursing training.

I was determined that I was going to be able to help other people so that other families wouldn't have to lose their father as well. At least that's what 14-year-old me had thought and wasn't going to be moved from.

CHAPTER TWO

The Stage is Set

'*The body weeps the tears the eyes never shed.*'
– Robert Bly

I found that I enjoyed nursing. Shift work, however, was tough. I would often find myself working night shifts. Sleep became something that was frequently in short supply. I struggled with my health throughout my training. On my way out one night, I was involved in a head-on collision with a drunk driver and was lucky to survive.

I escaped with a whiplash injury and a lot of bruises. The hospital where I was working gave me a soft collar to wear for six weeks and one physiotherapy session. I suffered for a long time with what might now be recognised as PTSD, or post-traumatic stress disorder, as a result. I had nightmares for years where I would wake in fright viewing looming headlights. It took many years before I could travel in a vehicle at night without feeling anxious.

During the months following the accident, I had a prolonged encounter with the Epstein-Barr virus – otherwise known as glandular fever. It's a common viral infection that usually resolves in a few weeks. I would be well for a while then relapse again. It took a long time to fully recover. Then one evening at work, while doing the medication round, I was attacked by a patient who almost succeeded in strangling me.

She was demanding a sedative and I was not able to give it to her. I was saved by one of my patients who repeatedly hit the call buzzer which brought the other staff running. It turned out she had a long history of similar behaviour and had been admitted under one of her many aliases. Police were called and she was taken away. I was not offered any counselling or assistance. I was instead told not to return to work until the bruising around my neck was gone as it would upset the patients.

In the lead up to my final exams, I was given special treatment by the rostering team. For three solid months, I cycled between night and day shifts. Week on, week off, having to study on top of it. I performed exceptionally well despite the disruption and was very happy with my results. Not long after, I developed pneumonia. I was extremely unwell with a partially collapsed lung. It took a long time to recover.

Despite the downsides, once I became a registered nurse I moved back to Canberra. I started in an endocrinology ward where we had a lot of patients with chronic health issues including diabetes. We were also the step down ward for patients who had suffered a heart attack to be rehabilitated before going home. I developed a keen interest in exercise as we used it to help our patients manage their blood sugar and gain confidence before discharge. From there, I moved fairly quickly into the coronary care unit.

On the day he died, my father had been found by the paramedics in ventricular fibrillation: an abnormal heart rhythm that was probably the ultimate cause of his death. I had this burning need to find out everything I could about the heart and why that might've happened. It was always at the back of my mind. My father was only 35 when he passed.

As a result, I was constantly pricking my ears up every time we admitted someone young. I would pay extra attention to what was going on for that person. The youngest patient I remember had a heart attack at 28. I was ever hopeful of finding the answer. The closest I came was that for some reason it happens in younger people and it is known as sudden cardiac death syndrome. I had to accept that. My mother, however was still looking for answers until the day she died. She could never let it go.

With what I know now, I believe this was actually very detrimental for her health. She could never accept that he was gone. She just didn't seem to find closure because she never got a reason. So, despite the fact that my mother had remarried four years after my father's death, she still didn't do well. Her new husband once told me that he felt like he was living in the shadow of a ghost. Some nine years after my father's death, she was diagnosed with acute myeloid leukaemia.

I remember that day well. I had just turned 23. Perhaps three months' prior, mum had accompanied me to Melbourne for a chance to do some Christmas shopping. I was attending an interview for a specialty course that I had applied for at a Melbourne hospital. She had seemed her normal self. She was following a special diet in an effort to lose weight on her doctor's advice. He had recommended it because she had been complaining of increasing fatigue.

Despite her continued complaints, her GP had not done even a basic blood test. I had her seek a second opinion from my GP. He referred her to a cardiologist because he thought that he could hear a slight heart murmur. It was the cardiologist who finally did the blood test. He phoned me at work and asked me to take mum to his office immediately.

I had to find her at the local TAFE college where she was studying for her independent real estate license. She must have known it was bad. In the waiting room, she made notes like 'arrange solicitor to update will.' We went straight from his office to the hospital where she had a bone marrow biopsy and a central line inserted for chemotherapy to commence asap.

Now I had plans, of course, to go on with my career – but what does every good daughter do? Especially when you are the eldest and you're conditioned to be a family carer. I moved back home, and put my plans on hold to care for my sisters and mother. Mum was really not inclined to accept the help of community nurses. After all, she had a daughter who was a nurse; why accept someone else? I kept my job in Coronary Care though, as I had a car loan to pay.

The doctors initially gave her only six weeks to live without any treatment. But with chemotherapy, perhaps she had a chance to live longer. There was a 50% chance that she might attain remission. So, she took that chance and had her first round of chemotherapy. It was really hard going and the bad news was, it didn't work. Then she was given one final chance: have another round of chemotherapy with an even lower likelihood for success. She took it and nearly bled to death as the hospital ran out of blood supplies. I was put on standby to fly to Sydney and be placed on a centrifuge machine. It's a way to quickly obtain platelets. She improved just in time, but it also didn't put her into remission.

Then we looked at the possibility of a bone marrow transplant. My sisters and I were all tested to see if we were compatible. Unfortunately, a donor couldn't be found. Mum was a fighter though and she told me, 'I'm not ready to die.'

I was looking after her at home as best I could, as well as working shift work in a very high-stress environment. It soon became too much for me. I was starting to crumble. I wasn't sleeping and had lost a lot of weight. I wasn't functioning at my best and something had to give. So, I quit nursing for a little bit and somehow managed to get myself a job at the High Court of Australia. Now, how does a nurse do that? Who knows? But somehow, I did.

I found myself working at the High Court as a library assistant. It was a really welcome change from the high-pressure hospital environment. As a public servant, I also had flexi time which made it so much easier to juggle accompanying mum to her appointments. It also allowed mum to start experimental low dose chemotherapy as I could give it to her at home.

I wasn't ready to give up on my career in health though. I saw this as a temporary move. I enrolled part-time in a degree in health education. I made it through the first semester before I chose to defer temporarily as mum's condition was unstable. Two years post-diagnosis, she was in and out of hospital as the treatment had stopped working.

It was at the court that I met my husband. When he asked me to marry him, my mother was not at all happy, to put it mildly. I reassured her that I wanted a long engagement but she suddenly had other ideas. She was in a rush to see me married before she died. I had three months to get organised from start to finish. Mum seemed to find a new energy and set the date for us.

I continued helping her to manage at home as best I could. She was in constant pain and on heavy medication. On her final Christmas day she asked me to assist her to take a shower. It was really her creating a private space to have a heartfelt conversation. She simply said, 'I'm ready to go, will you help me?' It came as a shock. I had to explain to her that all I could do was to ensure that she was treated with dignity and that I would do my best to keep her comfortable.

It was perhaps a week or two later that her pain became unbearable. I made the decision to call an ambulance and transfer her to the hospital. My sister was due to have her first child in three weeks. We arrived at the hospital and I needed to push to have her admitted for pain relief. The doctor in the emergency department was reluctant because she was already on a high dose of narcotics. I had to call in favours to make it happen.

Once she was under the care of the staff who knew her, they managed to relieve her pain. To do so, they had to infuse her with narcotics which helped but also caused her to hallucinate. One day I visited and she was seeing a beautiful baby boy. Her first grandchild, a boy, was born a week after her death. The next day she slipped into unconsciousness and died soon after.

I'd been married for almost a year when my mother passed away. Soon after, I discovered that I was expecting my first child. Not long after that, my husband, who was also very career-driven, took a temporary contract in Sydney. He was commuting back home on the weekends, leaving me still working at the court.

I was around six months pregnant when my grandmother, on my father's side, passed away very suddenly. I had only spoken with her on the phone a matter of days before. Her doctor had removed a melanoma on her arm. She had suddenly become very short of breath and sounded worried. I was very upset and unable to travel to her funeral. I sent two of my sisters instead. They were not warmly welcomed and I was later criticised for not attending.

Soon after, I was admitted to hospital having gone into premature labour at only 29 weeks' gestation. It was very stressful with my husband in another city four hours away. The staff prepared me for an emergency caesarean section. Back then, I knew that a baby born that early did not have fabulous chances of survival. Luckily, they managed to stop the labour. However, I was advised that I needed to remain in hospital to delay the birth as long as possible.

My husband suggested that it was better that I move to Sydney with him and have the baby there. It was arranged with my doctor to refer me to a doctor there. So, we moved to Sydney. I was 26 when our baby was born healthy and only two weeks early by emergency caesarean.

There I was: new mum, new city. I had lived there before but never ventured far outside of the hospital. This was just like being in a new city and it wasn't familiar. I didn't have my family or friends around at all. To top it off, my mother's parents were not coping. My mother had been an only child and they now looked to me for support.

My grandmother was admitted into a Sydney hospital in the hope that the program they offered could help with her depression. The hospital phoned and asked me to pick her up and take her for tests. I was unable to drive following my surgery and even then, I didn't know my way around. I had to decline. My grandfather pulled her out suddenly and took her home after only a few weeks.

Of course, I was an executor to my mother's estate. I was also guardian to my youngest sister who was still at school. I was very concerned for her. Once my son was six weeks old and I was allowed to drive, I travelled with him back to Canberra. We were sorting through my mum's house, getting it ready to sell. It was just too big to manage for my two sisters still living at home.

I invited my grandparents for afternoon tea as I wanted to see them before heading home the next day. Just before they were due to arrive my grandfather phoned and said, 'I'm sorry, grandma's not feeling well. Would you mind dropping in and seeing us tomorrow on your way home instead for morning tea?' So I reluctantly agreed. What could I do? She wasn't well.

My son was really fussy in the morning. It was a long drive back to Sydney by myself with a new baby. I decided not to stop by, instead heading straight home. I expected to have to return soon enough and I would see them next time.

I arrived back in Sydney, to be told by my husband that he'd received a phone call. My grandparents had been found that morning by a neighbour. They had double suicided. To realise that I was the one who was supposed to find them was devastating.

I was now the executor of two deceased estates. I had to arrange their funeral. They wanted to be buried back in South Australia, so we held a memorial service and they were buried alone. I had to juggle solicitors, and real estate agents, travelling back and forth with a baby in tow. To top it off, we moved four times in just over a year as well. I realise now that I didn't have time to grieve.

My second son was born not quite two years after the first, also by emergency caesarean section. I had a difficult pregnancy this time with extreme nausea and vomiting at times. I found that I was constantly exhausted. I remembered that during my first pregnancy I had a high iron level when they tested my blood. My doctor back then had told me to stop taking iron tablets. When I had informed her that I wasn't she had said that I must have been and just didn't realise it!

I had done my research and learned of a condition called haemochromatosis. I knew something was not right. I asked my doctor to test my iron again and it was even higher. He was not concerned and said, 'Vicki, just because you're a registered nurse you don't need to make more out of this than it is.' I kept feeling worse and worse. I again had to give up my work, by then as a community nurse. The nausea was constant and I was so fatigued at times that I could barely manage with two young sons.

I insisted on being referred to a specialist. He reluctantly referred me to a gastroenterologist and at the same time, told me that I should get out more. I should find a mother's group he said and offered me an antidepressant. The gastroenterologist glanced at my results and asked, 'where did you get all that iron from?' before putting them aside and telling me that I had irritable bowel syndrome. He was conducting an experimental treatment study that I could pay to join. I declined.

Eventually, I found a doctor who could pinpoint what was wrong: haemochromatosis. I had a genetic condition predisposing me to absorb too much iron. It was treated with many trips to the blood bank to donate blood. It was long and arduous but the only way to do it. With each venesection, a little iron was removed. I went weekly at first and then tapered off to monthly over a year or so. I had to take my boys with me when they were not at preschool.

It wasn't too bad as they enjoyed the treats that the staff gave them. I was told that I probably wouldn't be able to have any more children. The damage to my organs from the iron may have permanently affected my chances. Slowly, I started to feel like my old self again. I was attending the gym regularly and enjoying bike rides with my boys.

I had a new GP who was interested in alternative treatments. He had a heavy metal test that he invited me to take. It, of course, read high. He gave me a bottle of clear liquid to take a few drops in water every day. To this day, I don't know what was in it. Whatever it was, I have rarely needed a trip to the blood bank since. He moved back to his home country so I never got to ask him.

Once my boys were both at school, I started to think about a return to work. Then, out of the blue, having believed it impossible, I discovered that I was expecting my third child. Another emergency caesarean, this time on Melbourne Cup day. In case you haven't heard, it is known as the race that stops the nation.

It was not a good day. The anaesthetist was grumpy as he couldn't understand why I wanted to remain awake. 'For goodness' sake, it's her third! Why does she need to be awake?' he complained. Everyone was in a rush so that they wouldn't miss the race. The doctor had trouble with the delivery. It took four people pushing and pulling as I apparently had a lot of scarring from the previous surgeries. At one point I was scared that I would land on the floor. As I was being taken from the operating theatre, I heard the nurse ask for pain relief to be ordered. 'She doesn't need it,' said the anaesthetist.

I was of course in a lot of pain, but I was only given Panadol. The next day, I should have had all feeling back after the spinal anaesthetic. I couldn't feel my left leg though. It took a long time for some feeling to return. 35 years old, I couldn't control my foot properly and had to learn to walk all over again. I was prone to rolling my ankle as I could not feel it. I had a persistent slight limp. No one seemed overly worried though. It was probably just nerve damage from the spinal anaesthetic, my doctor said.

A year later we moved again. This time we had a two-level home. To reach the car, we had to go downstairs and through the backyard. I was rushing to get the boys to school as it was nearly Christmas and I was needing to shop. I had a specialist paediatric appointment to attend with my youngest on the other side of the city. I have no idea how it happened but I managed to fall down the stairs carrying a baby without hurting anyone but myself. They say that accidents and adverse events are more likely with things like moving, so I put it down to that.

I was still prone to the occasional fall but I didn't let it stop me. Once all my children were at school, at 41 I decided to move into a fitness career. I felt it was a really good use of my time. It fit in well with family life. It kept me fit and healthy and I was helping my clients achieve their goals. Life was good until one day, while I was out chatting with a neighbour, I was stung by a bee.

CHAPTER THREE

Down the Rabbit Hole

———•———

'When you resist, it persists.'

I remember pulling the sting out and making my way back upstairs. I must have been feeling a little bit woozy because I had lain down on the floor. I don't think I passed out, but I remember coming back into the reality of the room with my eldest son, who had recently completed his first aid certificate, saying, 'Are you okay, mum?' I remember saying something like, 'Yeah, I'm fine.' But I wasn't at all fine. I was dizzy, quite dizzy. The site of the sting was not only swollen, it had a big red line running all the way from my shoulder up the back of my neck.

Feeling no better after a few days, I went to the doctor. He thought that it was unusual enough that it should be checked out. He ordered some blood tests. When the results came back, they indicated that I had a moderate immune reaction to bee venom. I was then referred to an immunologist, who told me one more sting and I might not be so lucky. I had a potentially fatal problem. And beyond that, I might also react to a wasp sting in a similar way. There was also a jumping jack ant which also could create a problem, but they luckily were not common.

He wrote me a prescription for an EpiPen and said that I should carry it with me at all times. I asked what else could I do, as bees are everywhere. I was teaching an aqua fitness class at an outdoor pool and there were often bees that landed in the water. He told me that I should stop pretending to be a flower. I laughed because I didn't think that I did. 'Do you wear perfume?' he asked. I agreed that yes, I did sometimes. 'Well, stop it!' he said. 'And don't wear bright, colourful clothing. If you look and smell like a flower, you're more likely to attract a bee.'

Then he explained that I would need to start desensitisation shots. We would start at a very tiny dose and slowly build up. It would take three years but hopefully it would reduce the chance of a life-threatening reaction. He also decided to test me for any other allergies as I did suffer quite badly from hay fever at times. It showed that I was basically allergic to pollen from every single grass that grows on the planet as well as, of all things, the pollen from olive trees and related species.

It was decided that since we were going to be doing shots, we might as well add the pollens in as well. The injections had to be ordered from France. Once they arrived, I had to go back to the immunologist for the first dose in case I had an adverse reaction. I was fine. I then continued to visit my GP to have my shots. I had to wait for half an hour after the injection to make sure that I didn't have an adverse reaction, as each time the dose was slightly increased.

I only managed to keep up with the injections for perhaps 12 months. I had begun to experience joint pain and swelling. It started in my fingers. It got so bad that I couldn't use my hands. The immunologist put me on colchicine, a medicine commonly used for gout, in the hope that would ease the symptoms. It did not help. My joints became so painful that I couldn't get a good night's sleep.

My specialist said, 'We might have to stop the pollen as it might be overstimulating your immune system.' I agreed: pollen wasn't exactly life-threatening and could wait. But despite that, things got much worse. Even the cartilage between my ribs and breastbone and spine was inflamed. Sometimes it hurt so much that I was afraid to breathe. I tried everything. Out of desperation, I even bought a new mattress, hoping that it might help, but nothing seemed to make a difference.

The immunologist thought that it was possible that I might be developing a very rare autoimmune disease called relapsing polychondritis, where the immune system mistakenly attacks cartilage in the body. He prescribed me an anti-inflammatory that was lifesaving at the time. I was finally able to get some sleep. Pain relief gave me some hope that I would see further improvements. It couldn't have been more than a few months when it was suddenly withdrawn from the market.

Someone else taking it had unfortunately passed away due to liver failure. The TGA withdrew it as a precaution as reports of other patients with liver problems came to light. I felt a sort of desperation without it. As soon as I stopped taking it, everything hurt again. Knowing that I already had haemochromatosis, and that my liver was prone to potential problems, I went to my GP.

A blood test showed that my liver was in trouble. It was pure luck that the drug had been withdrawn. For all I know, I could have been the next fatality. I had none of the usual symptoms but my liver was not functioning normally. We decided that I should stop the bee desensitisation as well. I would just have to be extra careful.

Throughout this whole process, I had been carrying on with my fitness career. It had become more like fitness 2.0 though. I'd had to really change the way I was doing things, giving up personal training because I couldn't even pick up weights anymore to assist my clients.

I kept up with my aqua fitness and falls prevention for senior's classes, as I could still manage those. Fortunately for me, there are lots of ways to modify exercise for older people. Until one day I was teaching a class and I couldn't keep up with my 80-year-olds. What was going on? Now I had knee and shoulder pain and a crushing muscular fatigue. Not liking to let people down, I kept turning up. A lot of these people had problems like Parkinson's disease and heart conditions. If they could show up, surely I could too.

Most of my aqua classes were in rehabilitation pools. I worked with a lot of elderly people and people with disabilities. I even had a bilateral amputee coming to one of my classes. So, they were fairly easy going for me. It wasn't really so physically taxing as all I needed to do was stand on the edge of the pool and give them instructions. They had been coming to my class long enough to still receive a good workout. It was social for them as well and they looked forward to the Christmas party I organised for them at the end of the year.

I had kept one class that was still high-powered. It was held at night for people to attend after work. They were younger and they liked to exercise pretty hard. I enjoyed it too as sometimes I would join them in the pool. Water is a good low impact supportive environment and the cooler water was easy on my joints.

I had started noticing some unusual sensations afterwards as I dried off. Bending forward would cause a strange tingling sensation down my spine, ending with a feeling that a feather was tickling my leg. I had a friend who was a radiologist and he had once mentioned that anyone over 35 would show some degree of spinal deterioration on X-ray. I figured that was probably also true for me so I wasn't overly concerned. Eventually, I had to stop getting in the pool with them as it became too hard on me. I was only able to teach from the side of the pool.

Then one night, I remember feeling not at all well. I couldn't look at the lights as it hurt my eyes. I was dizzy: it was like after the bee sting all over again. So instead of standing up on the edge of the pool, I needed to sit on one of the diving blocks on the end of the pool and teach from there.

Even then my class participants kept asking, 'Vicki, are you okay? You don't look too good.' I assured them I was okay. I didn't feel 100%. Really, I was not okay. It was my favourite class though so I pushed through. I felt bad enough to visit my GP. After an examination he said to me, 'You have meningism.' That was something I had not heard of and it sounded serious.

The meninges are the outer covering of the brain. If that gets infected, you've got meningitis. That can be a serious problem sometimes requiring hospitalisation. Meningism, I was told, was inflammation often caused by a viral infection. Well, I had contracted what seemed to be a viral infection earlier in the year. It had left me feeling a bit flat, but that was months ago. Surely that couldn't be it. But he said to me, 'Look, you're overdoing it.

Unless you want long-term problems, you need to give yourself six months to really rest.' And so reluctantly, as it was almost the end of the year, I cancelled all of my classes.

I found replacement instructors and took six months off. It would mean starting again once I returned, because once you gave your classes away you did not get them back. I retained some private clients. I had trained in SCENAR therapy back when my pain was unbearable. It is an electronic device that works on similar principles to acupuncture, only without the needles. It was really helpful for my clients with injuries to aid recovery. I was going to be fine. Six months would be enough.

Once my six months was up, I gave out notice that I was available. I expected to have to wait but I was offered classes straight away. So, on my first day back, I had three classes back-to-back with a big commute in between. My fitness level had waned a bit over that time. They were aqua classes for seniors and it should not have been a big deal. I made it through the day, but it wasn't my best performance.

The next day I got up, and saw my kids off to school. I had a class to do later in the day, but I was just so worn out. Everything hurt again and I couldn't get off the couch. I had to phone in and say, 'I'm really, really, sorry. I don't know what's wrong with me, but I can't move. I'm not going to be able to make this class.' Actually, I never made it to another.

I thought I should seek out the help of a rheumatologist. Surely that was my next step. I would find some answers and be able to continue on. This doctor sent me for X-rays and blood tests. The X-rays were excruciatingly painful as I had to hold myself in very uncomfortable positions to get the right angle. Nothing conclusive showed. The blood tests showed that I had been infected with Ross River fever. It's an infection carried by mosquitoes and I had become unwell following a holiday in Queensland. That was consistent with the viral infection theory at least.

I was put back on an anti-inflammatory medication and more rest. 'You need to give it time,' I was told. So, I used my time productively, with further study, adding to my professional development in anticipation of returning to work. I still had a few SCENAR clients but I couldn't manage much else on top of looking after my family. By the time a year rolled around, I was even worse than when I first had sought help. I was packing on weight and I could barely manage to write with a pen. Simple things like making a coffee caused extreme pain in my fingers. It was time for another opinion.

I did a Google Scholar search and found someone who had published research on conditions associated with joints and haemochromatosis. It seemed logical to me that there would be a connection. An appointment was made fairly quickly with another rheumatologist and I had really high hopes that he was my answer. After more tests, he finally gave me a diagnosis: Serum-negative ankylosing spondylarthropathy (which he admitted making up to fit my symptoms). I met all but one of the criteria. I did not have the usual blood markers, but everything else fit.

So, I started on the medication that he prescribed but I soon developed really strange sensations in my feet. He advised me to stop the medication. He said it was unusual but that it could be a rare side effect. But things got much, much worse. I remember meeting a friend for lunch. Standing on the side of the road waiting to cross, I had asked her if someone was tunnelling nearby. My whole body felt like it was shaking, but she couldn't feel anything.

Then one morning I woke up and couldn't feel my legs properly up to my knees. My rheumatologist insisted I see a neurologist. I couldn't get an appointment quickly. By the time I saw him, I was struggling to walk. It felt like I was at sea. I felt sure that people would think I was drunk.

Just the week, before I'd taken my car for a service. Normally, I would walk a short distance to the local shopping centre and have a cup of coffee while I waited. But walking was a struggle. An old lady actually passed me with her little wheelie walker. If I could have moved faster, I almost would have asked her to let me have a seat on her walker, I was struggling that badly.

The neurologist didn't really feel that there was going to be anything much to find. He sent me for an MRI and some nerve conduction tests. I went back to see him some weeks later only to be told that at 47 I had multiple sclerosis. It's hard to describe how that felt. I remember asking if diet and exercise could help. He said no they would not but my past exercise had probably helped somewhat. 'Oh, and don't eat fried food,' he added.

I still had that feeling of being slightly unwell, like when you are coming down with something. Knowing that I had a persistent viral infection, I was worried about the recommended treatment. I expressed my concern only to be told 'there are no other options.' Basically, I was to have five massive intravenous doses of prednisone to shut down my immune system, as it was attacking me! Then I would take a high dose in tablet form and slowly taper off over six weeks before commencing further treatment.

I phoned a good friend of my parents who I had kept in close touch with. She knew someone with MS and would ask her advice. The advice was 'take anything they give you.' So, reluctantly, I agreed to have the infusions. I was assured that I would feel much better as they hooked me up to the first infusion. For a little while I did, the painful swelling in my joints improved, but following the fifth infusion I started to feel much worse.

I was miserable. A friend, who is a scientist in medical research, came to visit. He just looked at me shaking his head. 'You look really sick, it's a shame there is no hope for a cure,' he said. To top it off, I was having what can only be described as intrusive thoughts. I couldn't stop thinking about how I could end my life. The experience of losing my grandparents was enough to stop me though. There was no way I would put my kids through that.

Knowing that I needed help, I visited my GP. He adjusted the dosage schedule to wean off the prednisone quickly and safely. At my follow-up appointment with the neurologist, I was told that the latest MRI was not good. I was to start injectable medication and needed to have an MRI every six months. He wanted to keep a very close watch on what was happening. There were stronger medications that he could try and I would be able to access mobility aids when I needed them.

I had a nurse visiting regularly to make sure I was injecting properly. I had given more injections than I could ever count, just not to myself. I had such a bad tremor that I had to use a specially designed auto injector. I had to start using a walking stick. I was so slow that I couldn't keep up. Soon I couldn't go out, and felt that I couldn't do anything.

So eventually I caved in and got myself a mobility scooter, which at least allowed me to go out with my family, if only just to do normal things like visit the shopping centre. I still needed someone to move it for me, to put it in and out of the car, and put it together. I was by no means fully independent.

My nurse congratulated me for being so accepting of my condition. She asked me would I mind being featured as a story in the drug company's MS magazine. It was like being hit by lightning. 'Wait a minute, I'm not accepting this,' I thought. I was sick of missing out on life.

CHAPTER FOUR

The Line in the Sand

'Action is the foundational key to all success.'
– Pablo Picasso

A friend asked me If I had heard about the book, *The Brain That Changes Itself* by Norman Doidge MD. I had not and they recommended it. A soon as I could, I read it. In it, Doidge outlines how the brain has the capacity to rewire and grow and change. Now, this was contrary to everything that I'd learned in my nursing studies. We were taught that once there was damage to the brain, it was permanent. I had initially accepted that I would be limited to small, if any, improvements. This was inspirational and gave me renewed hope.

I devised my own rehabilitation exercise plan. Slowly but surely, I started to experience small improvements which were very encouraging. I found that the more I improved, the more I did. In turn the more I did, the greater the improvement. Little by little. Not anything especially earth-shattering, but encouraging nonetheless.

I started with the activities that limited my everyday existence. Something as small as standing without holding onto something seems inconsequential now, to stepping forward with my worst leg first. I started to implement strategies that I had used with past clients. A little trick that professional gymnasts use is to visualise.

Before they attempt a new routine, on say the uneven bars, they first play it through in their mind. By the time they actually physically perform it the brain has already formed the neural pathways. Our minds are the most powerful tool we have. We're capable of so much more when we learn to utilise them.

Soon after, I learned about the work of Professor George Jelinek. He is an Australian doctor who had also been diagnosed with MS. In fact, his mother had passed away with MS. He had been so determined to change his course that he took six months off work to do some intensive research. It paid off and he had halted the progression of his disease.

In the book, he detailed his recovery. He had devised a dietary and supplementation plan called the OMS program (Overcoming Multiple Sclerosis). His plan included meditation and mindfulness as well as exercise. So, I followed the diet because I figured, what have I got to lose? It's only food.

I found it was tough going at first. It was a very strict diet: vegan plus fish. No dairy, eggs or meat. The first thing I remember telling myself was that I could not give up cheese. It sounds stupid in hindsight. I had to remind myself that nothing tastes better than healthy feels. I wanted my life back. I needed to focus on that goal and commit 100%.

It's really hard to prepare meals when you can't stand for long. So, I bought a stool for the kitchen. I had to sit on it and do what I could. The fine motor control in my hands was limited so using a knife was a challenge. Adopting the diet meant a lot of vegetables and preparation. Fortunately, my kids were very good at helping me.

They were also happy to eat what I ate to save me having to double up on meals. It meant we had to find new recipes to try so that it didn't feel like we were missing out on too much. We made it fun and set challenges to find ways to recreate healthy versions of old favourites. My youngest took on the challenge for a school project and impressed their teacher so much that it was shared amongst the entire school.

Slowly, I started to see some tangible improvements. My walking was still painfully slow, like trying to drive with the handbrake on. Naturally, once you start to see some improvement, you want more. Being an avid researcher, I had hit the internet looking for anything else that I could find. It led me to a recently described condition called CCSVI.

Chronic cerebrospinal venous insufficiency: this was the discovery of an Italian vascular surgeon Dr. Paulo Zamboni. Decreased blood flow out is thought to slightly increase the pressure in the brain. Lesions typically seen in MS form in close proximity to blood vessels in the brain. He had devised a treatment that he had used to help his wife. She had suffered from the debilitating effects of MS. He had made life-changing improvements for her and I was determined to find out more about it.

I joined an online forum for MS patients. There was a CCSVI thread with patients worldwide. The majority were in America. Quite a few of them had received the treatment and were doing well. I didn't have any hope of making it to America. I eventually came across a group of MS patients here in Australia. Some of them had received the treatment here and were also seeing improvements.

They were holding an information evening in Melbourne which Dr. Zamboni was attending. This was an opportunity too good to miss. Also at the meeting was a doctor from Newcastle who was assisting patients with the diagnostic process.

I made an appointment to see Dr. Paul Thibault in Sydney as he was consulting occasionally there to make it easier for his patients. He asked me about my medical history, specifically infections. I remembered that I had pneumonia when I was a student nurse. He explained that certain bacteria can cause problems with blood vessels. He ordered an ultrasound study of the veins in my neck and found that I did, in fact, meet the criteria for CCSVI.

There was a small clinical trial being undertaken in Sydney and I was placed on the waiting list. After a couple of months, I received notice that I was next on the list. I completed the paperwork and sent it back. I was given the date and instructions for the day. It was to be an outpatient treatment with no hospital stay. I was all prepared when with very short notice everything was suddenly cancelled without explanation.

Undeterred, I was referred to an interventional radiologist in Melbourne. We had a phone consultation and based on my ultrasound results he agreed to help me. It was becoming somewhat controversial, however: Dr. Zamboni had unfortunately called the procedure 'liberation therapy.' It was being demanded by patients worldwide.

Neurologists saw red and were vehemently against it. It began to lose traction as it was dismissed as nothing more than placebo.

Despite this, I again travelled to Melbourne, this time for treatment. The procedure was done under a private arrangement, meaning it was completely at my expense. I was given absolutely no guarantees that it would help, but I had to try. Not having good blood flow out of the brain was surely not optimal. I knew of patients who had tried it and experienced no change. But nothing ventured, nothing gained.

The doctor had to access a large vein in my leg. It was very strange feeling the guide wire pass through my heart and up into my neck. I had seen many similar procedures whilst in coronary care. I had assisted our doctors to place stents in blocked arteries in the heart. Now I had a much better idea of what my patients had felt, except that their entry point was an artery with a higher risk of bleeding.

Once the catheter was in place, he injected a dye to outline the veins. There was a screen that enabled me to see reasonably well. My left internal jugular vein was completely blocked. So much so that nothing could be done to improve it. It was discovered that I had formed what is known as collateral circulation. The body is really clever and will create new blood vessels in an attempt to compensate. It's a little like a bypass; not as efficient, but better than nothing.

My right side wasn't much better. It was not completely blocked. After a couple of tries he managed to substantially improve the blood flow. He wasn't sure that it would hold, so I didn't expect too much. I did, however, have massive improvements.

The first thing I noticed was how much clearer my vision was. I had tried to maintain healthy scepticism going in. Being uncertain that it would help was, I suppose, my way of avoiding disappointment.

I was discharged after a few hours in recovery. There was a prescription for blood thinners to collect from the hospital pharmacy. It was down a long corridor. Normally that would have made me very dizzy but I was not even remotely affected.

I noticed later as we walked to the restaurant at our motel that my handbrake had been released. I was walking at a pace that was almost normal. With my new improvements I was able to give up the motorised scooter altogether. After a while, I found that I needed the walking stick less and less.

I was also taking antibiotics prescribed by my doctor in Newcastle. There were also a lot of supplements to take. He had adapted a protocol devised by Dr. David Wheldon, who sadly passed away in early 2021. His wife had developed MS and it was the result of his research. By following it, she had also recovered from her MS.

If you're interested in finding out more about that treatment, the ABC Catalyst program made a documentary called *MS Cure*. It features Dr. Thibault in Newcastle, Dr. Wheldon, his wife Sarah and myself. Although physical interventions for CCSVI are no longer available, there is still merit in the theory. If it were nothing more than placebo, why then would so many patients still be doing well? It also explores the infection theory in some depth.

Another documentary *The Living Proof* by Matt Embry is also worth viewing. He explores diet, CCSVI and other topics relevant to MS patients. Also worth exploring is the work of Dr. Terry Wahls, who also reversed her MS through diet and exercise. I will be forever grateful for each of their contributions.

From that point on, my improvement went from leaps to bounds. My life was finally back on track. I was able to walk longer distances consistently. My husband and I decided to travel overseas. We had three weeks in Europe. I had chosen a river cruise, having booked it prior to my treatment in Melbourne. Having become accustomed to my limited mobility, I had reasoned that even if I was not able to participate, at least I'd have a nice view. I actually managed to keep up with the walking tours, albeit with the slow group. I still needed the walking stick at times but we managed to have a great holiday.

We later went on to visit Lord Howe Island, where I even managed to snorkel with sharks! We also visited Vietnam and Cambodia where I climbed Angkor Wat. The more I took steps to challenge myself a little bit, the better I felt.

My neurologist, however, did not seem to see my improvement. I had not experienced a relapse or new changes visible on MRI for some time. Despite that, he wanted to put me on a new treatment that was associated with a rare but potentially devastating brain infection. I knew of other patients who had suffered irreparable damage as a result of it. He had initially indicated that it would only be necessary if the medication I was on became ineffective.

I questioned whether it was necessary given that my condition had now stabilised. He angrily told me that if I didn't accept his advice I was a fool and he couldn't help me! I sought a second opinion, only to be told that everything I had been doing was rubbish and to stop it. This new neurologist wanted me to start on another new treatment despite telling me that my MS was possibly now benign or burnt out.

Life for me was improving to the extent that I was itching to get back to work. I didn't want to go back to fitness or nursing. I knew that I still had a lot to offer and could help others. I needed to build on my past experiences. So, I chose health coaching. I was planning to launch my new business when out of the blue, my marriage came to an end.

It was not something that I could have foreseen. The circumstances surrounding it were quite traumatic. I knew that I needed to pay really close attention to my health. I had come so far and there was no way I wanted to risk going backwards. It took me a little while to regather my thoughts. I still had my two youngest living with me and they had not yet completed their studies.

I really needed to look after myself first if I was going to be there for them. I knew that in the past, I hadn't always done that. So, there was one thing that I knew I hadn't paid attention to when I followed Dr. Jelinek's OMS program. I had neglected to engage well with mindfulness and meditation. Back then it had seemed a little unnecessary and perhaps a bit woo woo.

I had justified it with what's the point in sitting down for 20 minutes, doing nothing, putting all thoughts out of your head. That didn't make sense to me then. But now, I knew I had to do something. You can't look after anybody else unless you look after yourself first, that much is clear. And like it or not, I was guilty of not always putting myself first throughout my life.

I searched for a meditation that would work for me. I had what is commonly referred to, in meditation circles, as monkey mind. Trying to put all thoughts out of your mind was like saying, 'Think of everything that you can all at once.' I just couldn't shut it off.

I had come across a company called Mind Valley, thanks to the power of Google retargeting. They sold an audio meditation program called Binaural Beats. It was music engineered to help you go into a meditative state without even trying. It actually worked. It had a really nice calming effect on me. Now, because I'd signed up with for one of their products, I was on their email list.

Into my inbox popped a masterclass by a hypnotherapist. I had been considering a hypnotherapy course and had one on my shortlist. So, I attended the rapid transformational therapy (RTT) masterclass. It was a massive 'aha!' moment. Not necessarily for me personally at that time. Rather, it conjured up memories of clients that I had worked with, patients that I nursed years ago and family members. It made so much sense. It explained some of the behaviours that had previously confounded me.

This could really help my clients who were stuck. Over the years, I had seen so much self-sabotage. My clients would be doing so well and all of a sudden give up; particularly those with chronic conditions like pain, excess weight and more. It was as if asking them to let it go was akin to them chopping a limb off. They just couldn't do it.

I started the training. I was gearing up to see my own clients and I had never asked anyone to do anything that I would not do myself. I learned a lot about human behaviour. I discovered that I had been pushing through without listening to my body. That it was related to the way that I'd been brought up as a child and the experiences that I had.

I had been curious about a particular method used to instruct the body to make certain changes, like heal a broken bone quickly. I still had areas of numbness and walked with a bit of a limp. I couldn't feel my big toe on my left foot very well at all. There were still little niggly reminders and I wanted to see if it could help. I put a call out to my fellow students.

I had my first real hypnotherapy session. As was my practice, I maintained a healthy degree of scepticism. I asked my colleague to instruct my nervous system to rewire itself. She went further and explored my relevant beliefs from childhood with me. The results were better than I expected. The feeling that I had lost in my foot 20 years before came back. My slight limp disappeared completely.

Once I graduated, I started to see my own clients. I found that because of my background, I was starting to attract people with health issues. Complex problems need multifaceted solutions. Most of my hypnotherapy clients were searching for new ways to tackle old problems, like struggling to lose weight for years without success or dealing with long-term anxiety and pain.

Some needed help with adapting to new situations. I had one elderly gentleman who had been a competition tennis player in his younger days. He had been so fiercely competitive that he had caused himself serious injuries. He needed to dial down that drive so that he could enjoy a social game of lawn bowls.

I wanted to add further to my knowledge of nutrition. I took a course in nutrition coaching. There was nothing wrong with it but it left me needing to know more. My sister had phoned and asked me what I knew about kidney stones. Her son had multiple stones in both kidneys and was in a lot of discomfort. She had almost lost a kidney to a stone herself. I did some research.

It led me to Julie Matthews, the founder of the Bio Individual Nutrition Institute and author of *Nourishing Hope for Autism*. Julie is a nutritional consultant, well known for her work in children with autism. Through this research, she discovered that food is an important factor to consider in autoimmune conditions as well. Food can be nourishing or problematic depending on your individuality.

I completed her Bio Individual Nutrition practitioner training. Through the course of my studies, I identified some of my own food sensitivities, allowing me to further tweak my diet and improve persistent joint issues. Ironically, sometimes the foods we crave cause us the most problems.

PART TWO

CHAPTER FIVE

On the Merry-Go-Round

'No problem can be solved from the same
level of consciousness that created it.'
– Albert Einstein

If you want to get well you need to be committed. There may be a lot of things that you need to change. I don't mean just following the doctor's orders – and I'll tell you why.

While modern medicine has overcome a lot of hurdles, there are limits to what it can do. Don't get me wrong: if I have an emergency medical situation, like a heart attack or a stroke, I really want medicine to come to my aid. If I have been involved in an accident or had some other physical trauma, I have a better chance of survival now compared with even a few years ago.

These days, doctors can do amazing things to put people back together and heal them from incredible physical traumas. They can sometimes remove bullets from brains without causing major damage. Modern treatment for stroke can now limit the amount of damage done so that patients have a better chance to live a normal life. A heart attack can be stopped in its tracks or even prevented with the timely placement of a stent. The medical leaps and bounds in recent years have been nothing short of amazing.

There's a catch when it comes to chronic medical conditions. For the first time in history, the average life expectancy in America has gone backwards. They are one of the largest populations on Earth, so the observational study size is immense. This is not just a random finding. Our modern lifestyle is catching up with us and dragging us backwards. Diet has a lot to do with it but it's not the full picture.

Doctors are limited in what they can do. They don't have X-ray vision like Superman. They can't always look into the body and see exactly what is happening. There is no magic crystal ball that can predict every future problem. They only have what tools they have, plus the collective knowledge gained from experience and research.

To put it in perspective, in order to treat us they have to arrange things in an order that makes sense. The human body is so complex that the knowledge has been arranged a little bit like books in a library. You know, if you need to find a particular book on a particular subject you can look up its location. Librarians use a cataloguing system, so that it's easy to find.

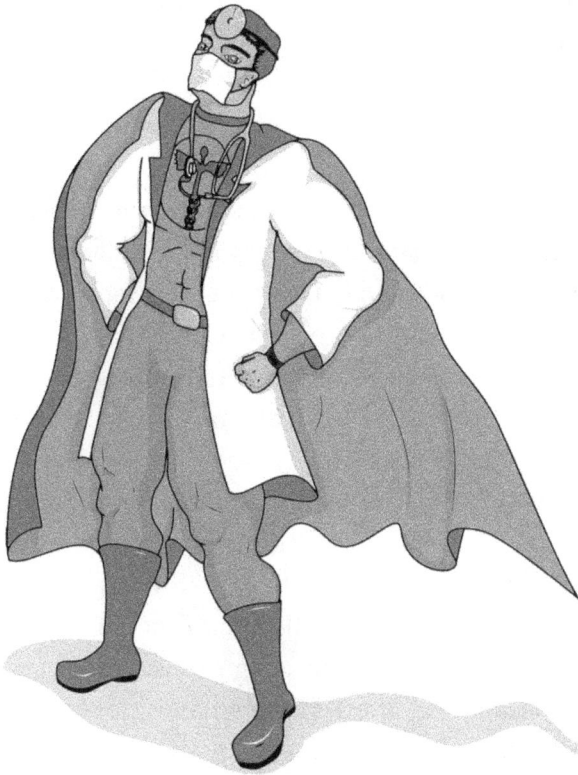

Medicine has tried to do a similar thing. The body is catalogued into systems. The lungs are the respiratory system, the heart and blood vessels are the cardiovascular system etc. Diagnosis is then made through a process of elimination called differential diagnosis. What that means is the doctors basically have a checklist of certain signs and symptoms. They call it diagnostic criteria. Added to that are the results from testing that offer known parameters.

There needs to be a specified number of criteria in a certain category to meet the diagnostic criteria. To put it another way: if it looks like a duck and sounds like a duck, then it's probably some sort of duck. Digging a little deeper should identify the type of duck and so on. That has limitations, of course, but it's been that way since the early days when doctors first started learning about the body.

It doesn't always look at the cause. Not everybody's condition is caused by the same thing. And no two people with the same diagnosis will have exactly the same symptoms or presentation of disease. The same treatment may or may not work for different people with the same diagnosis. MS is a very good example of this. It would be unlikely, if you picked two people with MS, to witness exactly the same signs, symptoms or responses to treatment. Unfortunately, doctors can only do their best with what they've been given.

I'm pleased to say that things are starting to change. There are reasons to hope that we are on the verge of a paradigm shift in medical care. Over the course of the last 20 years, I have seen more and more doctors stand up and talk about functional and integrative medicine. Instead of just categorising disease, they are looking at the body as a whole and questioning what might be the root cause of xyz condition. Recently I have seen an extension of this with some doctors now prescribing lifestyle medicine, including advice like go out and enjoy nature, meditate or join a yoga class.

There is a new movement calling themselves Lifestyle Medicine Practitioners. I recently attended their first online summit aimed at educating doctors on the benefits of prescribing lifestyle medicine. They advocate for the benefits of nature, good food and incorporating wellness coaching into medical practice. I have high hopes that they will shape the future of health care.

Until then, we need to take the initiative to inform ourselves and, in the process, educate our doctors. Never underestimate the power of planting a seed. Simply asking your doctor, 'Do you prescribe lifestyle medicine?' could help to set the wheels in motion. If nothing else, it opens up room for a conversation. It's important to build a relationship with your doctor.

You need to be comfortable with opening up, but also with standing up for what you want. Take a partner or friend for support if you need to. If you don't feel comfortable with what it is that they're offering, don't be afraid to ask the hard questions.

- Is this a medical emergency?
- Do I need to decide straight away?
- What complications might there be?
- What are the alternatives?

It is said that it can take up to 30 years for new practices to be adopted in medicine. I would be the first to admit however, as a traditionally trained nurse, I was sceptical the first time I learned about a holistic GP. The fees were very high compared with a regular GP and I didn't see the value. That was around 20 years ago. Having had my own journey, my views have changed. I regularly attend online conferences and summits to keep myself informed.

I follow a lot of these trailblazers on social media. I recently read a post by a young British doctor lamenting that she was restricted to 'pharmageddon' by the National Health Service (NHS). She understands the importance of lifestyle but her hands are tied. She's right: there's a pill for every ill, and doctors are encouraged to prescribe according to the diagnosis that they've made. Health care has become sick care and it's a multibillion dollar industry.

But here's the rub. Medications are prescribed for their desirable effects. They also come with undesirable effects that are referred to as side effects. An unspoken effect of a lot of medications is that they can rob the body of essential nutrients. This in turn can increase the risk of further problems.

A well known example of this is with statins. They are a class of drug prescribed to reduce cholesterol and so purport to reduce the risk of heart attack. It has been well documented that statins reduce the levels of a powerful antioxidant CoQ10. Ironically, CoQ10 supplementation has been shown to improve a range of cardiovascular symptoms. It also protects cholesterol from harmful oxidation and is important for muscle health and development, and it begs the question whether supplementation alone would suffice.

Hopefully by now, most doctors would know to supplement CoQ10 for their statin patients. I could go on with many more examples as there is barely a medication that does not have a negative impact on another function in the body. The body requires B group vitamins, including magnesium, calcium, zinc, vitamins A, C, D and E and many other nutrients to perform even the most basic functions.

It's important to understand that medications can increase your risk of other problems. I used to see this all the time when I was nursing patients with chronic medical conditions who were taking multiple medications. A medication would be prescribed for a problem, but the side effects of that medication, for example, might cause other problems. To deal with those, they would be prescribed another medication.

It could be the one thing that your doctors don't fully understand. Either they're not educated or they don't have the time to learn. Ask any doctor how much time was spent on nutrition in medical school. Most of them will tell you not much. It's also not obvious that it's happening behind the scenes as it can take a long time to show signs. The liver, for example, can struggle on for quite a while before signs of trouble show up in a blood test.

A lot of functions in the body are going on automatically. We're not aware of things like our liver detoxifying and processing. The liver has the job of producing glutathione. It is known as the master antioxidant. It is produced by the same pathway in the liver that breaks down many medications and toxins. While it is busy doing that, glutathione levels drop, inflammation increases and we get symptoms. Your doctor may feel the best choice is another medication. There are many more examples of this.

Doctors, at least here in Australia, are one of the most regulated professions. They are monitored not only by the government but also their own Medical Associations, on both state and federal levels. GPs are also a part of a local network. Specialists are admitted to colleges. They are expected to attain certain outcomes for their patients. At the same time, they are monitored for over-servicing so that they don't order unnecessary tests or see too many patients!

A lot of education is provided by drug company representatives. They are employed to visit doctors, tell them about new medications and educate them regarding their use. They leave samples to make it easy to start patients on a particular treatment. They are so keen to persuade that a busy doctor might unknowingly be influenced by them.

I remember a visit to my coronary care unit by a drug company representative. Their mission was to persuade us to use their 'new' drug over the one that our doctors were prescribing. There was little to no difference between the two medications' efficacy except for company profit margins. Theirs was newly patented, and ours was older, out of patent and therefore cheaper.

They came armed with a tray of French pastries to share amongst staff while providing education around their product. Ironically, the pastries were laden with fat and sugar in an area where all of our patients were prescribed a low-fat diet. We were also located adjacent to the diabetic ward.

Around the same time, during a visit to a GP, you would find drug company-branded toys in the waiting room, branded coffee mugs on the desk and even a branded pen to sign with on payment. Laws have thankfully been changed to limit this questionable practice. There is nothing to stop a company from sponsoring events like seminars though.

My first neurologist regularly had lunch with the nurse from the drug company that produced my medication. There was nothing to stop her paying for lunch, I imagine. On top of that, we are influenced every day by subtle marketing. Product placement in movies is one example. There are pictures in magazines, on the back of the bus and almost everywhere we turn. Why would a busy doctor be any different?

Back in the 1970s, governments gave medical research over to the big pharmaceutical companies. Most research is now funded by the very companies that stand to profit from the products that they develop. Studies only need to show that a medication performs just slightly better than placebo. A placebo is a sham treatment, or sugar pill, given to randomise a double-blind study.

If it's not profitable, it's not studied, which means that a lot of potential research isn't performed. Potentially good treatments can be shelved if they are deemed not profitable enough. This is outlined quite well by Colin T. Campbell in his book, *The China Study*. I would also recommend watching *The Living Proof* by Matt

Embry. In it, he outlines how pharmaceutical companies control funding within even charitable organisations like the MS Society.

Most other research comes via universities and privately funded research foundations. There is a lot of competition for limited government funding. There are many PhD and master's students contributing to research as well. It is easy to search on PubMed and find thousands of references to research on any topic.

Sometimes the only way off the path you are on is to find an alternative. This involves some work. There might be roadblocks or other obstacles in the way. One of the most empowering things you can do is explore, learn and take action.

CHAPTER SIX

Environment Matters

—————————— • ——————————

'Even the smallest changes in our daily routine can create incredible ripple effects that expand our vision of what is possible.'
– Charles F. Glassman

We live in a really exciting time at the moment. Medicine is starting to move towards the concept of holistic health. Holistic health is not a new idea, but it's thought of as being kind of 'new age-y.' In fact, it's been around for a long, long, long time. There are many proverbs or quotes that refer to the concept of a whole body. That is: everything that we do think or say, has an immediate and lasting effect on our health.

Some examples are:

'Health is a state of complete physical, mental and social well-being, and not merely the absence of disease and infirmity.' – World Health Organisation, 1948

'The doctor of the future will give no medicine, but will instruct his patients in the care of the human frame, in diet and in the cause and prevention of disease.' – Thomas Edison, 1902

'If we could give every individual the right amount of nourishment and exercise, not too little and not too much, we would have found the safest way to health.' – Hippocrates, ~ 400BC

Our body is the most incredible machine. It has the capacity to self-regulate, heal itself, to grow, to change and adapt. Unless we're faced with extremes, we don't even notice environmental changes like temperature. We don't know that all these things are going on behind the scenes as our body just tries to maintain a state of balance, known as homeostasis. It does this in such a way that it can just kind of cruise along on autopilot and conserve resources. A lot of things have to happen in the background that we're not even aware of.

We are producing new cells all the time. Different parts of our body completely renew themselves at different rates. The cells that line our gut are renewed every four days. The cells in your liver are capable of renewing and, to a certain extent, it is even possible to regrow if part of it is lost. This is only if the load placed on the liver is not excessive or persistent. Your liver performs around 500 processes that are essential for survival.

We make new blood cells when the old ones have fulfilled their use and are filtered out and broken down by the spleen. We are the ultimate recyclers. The body reuses what it can and only gets rid of what's no longer any use. It does this through a process called autophagy, mainly in your liver. It breaks down proteins to amino acids, the most basic building blocks, to be used to build new proteins. So, the liver is really the powerhouse of the body. If your liver fails, everything fails. The liver also regulates our energy, storing excess glucose as glucagon for later use.

It takes a lot of energy to run the body. It's not only our activity that drives our energy needs, it's our emotions. Are we happy? Are we excited? Are we sad or angry? They all use different levels of energy. They all have a different effect on the body and how the body functions as the abnormal body tries to normalise over time. So, why does the body fail? We have the capacity to recover from infection and heal from physical injury, but what happens when there's too much demand on resources? The body just has to prioritise.

It has to first provide energy to the things that are most important, which are keeping us alive. And so other things get pushed to the back and not given the attention that they really deserve. Lifestyle or functional medicine looks to what things we're doing in our day-to-day life that are having an impact to find out what's putting that extra load on the body.

Because everything we think and do is having an impact, it's up to us to choose. What is it that we can do to limit our exposure to the things that cause that extra load on the body? There are things like toxins in our environment, even simple things that you don't even think about every time you buy that nice smelling laundry detergent, shampoo or cleaner for your kitchen bench tops. The chemicals that create that lovely lemony smell are particularly toxic.

The body has to do what it can to eliminate those toxins because they will cause us damage. So, while your body's busy getting rid of all those environmental insults, it can't be focusing on what it really needs to do, which is rest and repair.

Take simple steps by having a look at what's in your laundry cupboard, under the sink or in your bathroom cabinet. Start by removing what you can and swapping for better, more environmental, alternatives. Try simplifying things down to products that won't cause any harm. Take time to read your labels: if you can't pronounce it, it's definitely not good for you. Just by choosing organic you can remove pesticide levels in the body by up to 80% in a few weeks.

We're also surrounded by environmental toxins that we absolutely can't do anything about: from the paint on your walls, to the carpet on the floor, to the foam in your mattress and your couch. They're all full of things like flame retardants and stain resistant fabric protection. They are off-gassing and releasing chemicals into the air.

These are all toxic to us. We don't feel them. We don't see them. So, we don't know they're there, but little by little, they're adding to the toxic load that your body has to deal with. Your liver's working overtime trying to deal with all of these insults that are part of our modern world.

Start by removing what you can. You don't have to do it all at once. Some of these things, like cookware, are expensive but they expose us to chemicals and increase that overall burden. Swap out what you can. If you have a pan that you use most, consider replacing it and choose something better. If you wouldn't eat it, consider whether you should use it or put it on your body.

It's encouraging to see that as people vote with their wallets, manufacturers are stepping up. You can now buy fluoride and sodium lauryl sulphate free toothpaste. There are many personal care products that are free of known contaminants. You can find laundry detergents and cleaning products available with non-toxic ingredients. Be careful with the organic label though: it only has to amount to 1% of the total ingredients to qualify.

Remember, you have probably been accumulating toxins for a long time. The sooner you cut yourself some slack the better. Going slowly will allow your body some time to adapt.

Some things to start swapping out:

- Plastics – they all leach hormone-disrupting chemicals
- Non-stick cookware – older products might be toxic, but studies are inconclusive
- Chemical cleaning products
- Artificial fragrances – scented candles, air freshener, perfumes
- Aluminium – some cookware, deodorants
- Parabens and preservatives in skin care products
- Mercury – older dental fillings, some seafood
- Paints – choose low VOC (volatile organic compound)
- Fire retardants in clothing
- Exposure to vehicle exhaust
- Pesticides – conventionally grown food, flea and lice treatments

If these insults continue, damage can occur as the body adapts. Dis-ease becomes chronic as we try to stay in balance. Our bodies can compensate for our poor food choices, environment and other insults for a while. If adverse conditions continue for long enough, the body will just do its best to balance with what it's got. It will struggle on even when it is under assault and under-resourced. This is how chronic disease really can take hold and it creeps up. We don't even know that it's happening.

It is said that if you place a frog in a pot of water and slowly raise the temperature it will remain while it slowly boils to death. We're not frogs but not so dissimilar. We will never notice a decline if we don't pay attention.

My body was trying to tell me for a long, long, long time that things weren't right. I was so busy dealing, but not dealing, with my emotions. Due to the busy-ness of my everyday life I wasn't paying attention. I did not understand the concept of putting myself first. My body did its best to just keep going. It wasn't until things reached critical mass that I could no longer ignore my symptoms. And then my diagnosis was made based on those symptoms.

Genetics

The journey wouldn't be complete without talking about genetics. Now, a lot has been said about genetics since the early 1990s, when the human genome project was started. Of note, the aim was to find new drug treatments. A number of companies have sprung up where you can actually test your own genetics. It's remarkably easy and relatively cheap, but what does it all mean?

There's still not a lot known about what all of our genes do. Some of them have been well studied, others not so much. We have 23 pairs of chromosomes that contain our genes. Each pair makes up a double strand known as DNA. It contains the information, or instructions, on how to make up all the components in our bodies. At the basic level, it's really the instruction manual for our body: from how to make individual cells and organs, whether or not you're going to have blue eyes or brown eyes, right down to how to make the enzymes that digest our food. Every process has instructions contained in our DNA and it is very individual.

There's a lot of our DNA that science doesn't know if it even has a role. It's been labelled as junk DNA or, more recently, dark DNA. Basically, scientists don't know what it does or why it's there, but that might change in time.

Coming back to what we do know, our genes are made up of single nucleotide polymorphisms or SNPs. They are comprised of four amino acids: (A)adenine, (C)cytosine, (G)guanine and (T) thymine. Identified by these four letters, they contain the blueprint for the function each one performs. It is most likely how to make a particular protein, which is often an enzyme.

They can have a common or wild type, or a variation. DNA is constantly making more copies of itself and does so with remarkable accuracy. Occasionally a small change occurs – say a G is swapped to a C – and is seen as evolution. Some of these changes are seen as more important than others.

One of the more common is known as MTHFR, which stands for methylenetetrahydrofolate reductase. It is an enzyme that sits in the middle of a number of complex biochemical processes collectively known as the methylation cycle. It is known to have variations that can alter how well the enzyme functions. Around 40% of the population is thought to have a level of reduced function as a result. Enter the newly revitalised kid on the block: the supplement company.

Supplements are not completely new. Vitamin C has been available as a supplement since the 1970s. It was a common addition to the breakfast table. I remember orange-flavoured chewable vitamin C as a child. Then along came high dose B vitamins that dissolve in water as a fizzy drink, and their highly successful marketing. Savvy companies have told us about all the things we need to supplement for. We need them to have healthy skin, hair and nails. How did we ever manage before? The choices are endless.

The process of methylation goes on in every cell so it is vital. Depending on your particular variant you may not convert vitamin B12 and/or vitamin B9, folate, into the form required for homocysteine to be converted to methionine as efficiently. Have your eyes glazed over yet? I warned you it was complex. The bottom line is a number of processes may be compromised, or not.

A lot of emphasis has been put on it because many practitioners, doctors and scientists seized upon it as the answer to the world's problems. As did the supplement companies. By calling it a mutation they were able to generate a whole new industry. There are more brands of methylation supplements than I could ever count.

MTHFR is really just the tip of the iceberg when it comes to how your body functions. Methylation is at the centre of everything. It drives how the body reproduces cells, detoxifies and how it produces energy. A lot of focus has been placed on, 'Oh, I've got bad genes.' With the exception of a few, there is no such thing as bad genes. You just have what you have and whether or not those genes are turned on or turned off is really dependent on your environment.

Genetics load the gun, environment pulls the trigger

What are you thinking right now? What emotions are you feeling? That's right, it's not just environment, even your thoughts have an impact. You can actually turn genes on and turn them off. So even if you have a 'bad' or not optimal set of genes, eating well, living well, being happy and getting good exercise can keep those genes functioning at their best, so that you're not as compromised as you might think.

On the flip side, you can have a perfect set of genes that should be functioning optimally. By making poor food choices, not sleeping, thinking poor thoughts and being exposed to environmental toxins, your genes can be performing worse than someone who's got a potentially bad set. So, it's really not the be all and end all, but it's worth taking note that everything that you do has an impact.

Some science suggests that gene expression starts in the womb. Something else to consider is the egg that you came from existed before your mother was born. It is thought that these epigenetic changes could be permanent and even if not it might take up to seven generations to undo any adverse changes.

I was very interested in my genetics when I first heard that I could test it myself. Having lost both my father and mother at early ages, and knowing that both of my natural grandfathers died of lung cancer, it seemed important. Having hereditary haemochromatosis myself made me extra curious, I suppose.

I don't know what I was expecting to find. It was quite early on in genetics when you could first order your own analysis. It wound up taking me around six years of research to figure out the basics. I had to read everything that I could find and even then, it wasn't until I came across Dr. Ritamarie Loscalzo, founder of the Institute of Nutritional Endocrinology, that I gained further understanding. Attending her SHINE (Scientific and Holistic Investigation of Nutritional Endocrinology) conferences and trainings allowed me to gather most of the pieces.

I now know where my potential weaknesses lie. Some of them I cannot ignore as they could be quite significant for me. I have multiple charts outlining the functions of major SNPs. That's my curiosity satisfied. All I really needed was to focus on everything that I am covering in this book. If you are curious, by all means do your own test. You do, however, need to be prepared to find something very motivating!

CHAPTER SEVEN

Mind Your BS

———————————•———————————

'Whether you think you can, or think you can't – you're right.'
– Henry Ford

From the moment we're born, our mind is working to keep us safe. It does this by forming memories around the things that we experience. This is to ensure that if we have the same or similar experiences again we can act swiftly if we sense danger. This dates back to our early existence when the risk of death from tigers and other similar threats was very real. So, our brains have developed a system to quickly determine if we're safe or need to act.

One theory has divided the brain into three parts, dubbed the triune brain. First, is the primitive or reptilian brain. It is common to nearly all species and manages all the basic systems required to live. Take a crocodile for example. They just need to stay safe and find food.

We are born with just the bare minimum needed to survive. Once we are born the brain develops quickly. Now the second brain, known as the limbic system or mammalian/emotional brain, comes into play. This allows us to form social connection and empathy. Both the reptilian and mammalian brains form what we understand as the subconscious mind. It is responsible for over 90% of the brain's activity.

There is a lot of growth going on: new brain cells called neurons appear and connections are being made. Our third brain, or critical thinking brain, is developing too. This is our conscious mind. It comprises around 7% of our thoughts. We learn to walk, talk, feed ourselves and begin to interact with our surroundings. This is when we start to develop our belief system, or BS.

Studies have shown that children, up until about the age seven, are in a state of alpha brainwave. We have four main wave types that can be detected by EEG. They are beta, meaning awake with a normal level of alertness. In the alpha state we are relaxed, calm and aware but not thinking. Theta is a state of deep relaxation, such as in meditation, and delta is a deep, dreamless sleep state.

Children, as they're experiencing life, are basically absorbing everything that's going on around them. It's a bit like running on autopilot. We all do it throughout our days. Remember when you learned to drive a car – it was hard at first. After a while you could do it without thinking. Now, you can carry on a conversation, listen to the radio, all while planning what to have for dinner and still get home safely.

Young children don't yet have a lot of higher conscious thinking, let alone experiences to measure new things against. So, the mind does its best to categorise things with the knowledge that it's got. As experiences are filed away as memories, they are catalogued. We store both enjoyable and unpleasant or unsafe experiences for future reference.

It's efficient. Every time we come across something new or unfamiliar, we run it through the same process. Is this safe? Will this harm me? Will I enjoy it? If the answer is yes, it's safe: great, let's do this. If not, oh no, there's a problem; we react and avoid. So, to put this into practical terms, the beliefs we form can hold us back or propel us forward.

If you've had adverse experiences as a child, you can have this programming deep down in your subconscious mind. Through its filters, it's running every new experience that you want to take on. And if it finds that they might be dangerous or not in your best interest, it'll do its best to avoid it even if it means sabotage. It can also do its best to make the things that we believe to be true become reality for us. So, if you've had an experience prior to age 18, it could fit into a category known as ACEs or adverse childhood experiences. I have listed a few below. If you answer yes to any of these there is a good chance that you formed some beliefs attached to them.

- Did an adult ever intimidate, insult or humiliate you?
- Did an adult push, slap or grab you? Were you injured or marked?
- Growing up, did you often feel that you were unimportant or not loved?
- Were you made to wear dirty clothes, or felt you didn't get enough to eat or were otherwise neglected?
- Was a household member depressed or mentally ill? Or did a household member attempt suicide?
- Did a household member regularly drink or take drugs? Were they too incapacitated to care for you or take you to the doctor if needed?

- Were your parents separated or divorced?
- Was your mother often subjected to physical violence?

I had formed beliefs that mental health help was not of any value. I watched my grandmother go through a mental health system her whole life. It ended really badly despite all efforts to help her. They actually made her life a living hell. Well, that was how I saw it. Maybe that's how she saw it, I don't know. Perhaps that is also why I didn't think to seek grief counselling.

We can also form beliefs around enjoyable experiences. Believe it or not, even something enjoyable can cause problems in later life depending on the belief that we attach to it. I had a client, an older man who was having trouble eating healthy food, even though he knew he should. He was turning to all sorts of comfort foods and his doctor had warned him that he was on the path to self-destruction. We explored his beliefs around that.

As a two-year-old child with a broken leg he had memories of cuddles with his mum and lots of treats. Around the same time, he had memories of sitting in a dark room alone being forced to finish his vegetables. We were able to shift his beliefs around food by focusing on what he really wanted. When we focus on what it is that we want, our mind is compelled to make it happen because it wants to keep us happy.

The good news is that we can change our perception. In the same way that neuroplasticity allows the function of a damaged part of the brain to be assigned to another part we can rewire our thought patterns. We can update our subconscious programs just like we can update the operating system of a computer. Neurons that fire together then wire together. We need to ask ourselves: what are the beliefs that are holding us back?

In my experience there are some common to all of us. Not receiving care and attention can cause us to believe we are not lovable. If our past experiences have caused us to form the belief that no matter what we do we can't succeed, then we may believe that it's not worth trying. Or if our past experience has been that no matter how hard we try we're not good enough, then we might give up because we believe we're not good enough. Or we can form the belief that something is not available to us, and have thoughts such as, 'It might work for them but it won't work for me.'

This can relate to anything in life from academic achievements to employment and relationships and so on. So, what about chronic disease? If our past experience has been that members of our family or people that we knew didn't do well with chronic disease, we might form the belief that no matter what we do, we're not going to do well either. Particularly if our focus is directed there when our doctors question our family history. That can link back to the belief that it's in our genes.

Not all of us will have negative beliefs. Do you know someone who's actually done better than expected? My own mother was a classic example. She was given six weeks to live, but declared that she wasn't ready. She survived for nearly three years, way beyond what her doctors expected.

There were times when they couldn't understand how she was still alive. They'd be looking at her blood test results and asking me, 'Vicki, how is this possible?' I think it was possible because she simply wasn't prepared to give up. She believed that she could go on. She wanted to go on and her body was responding to the directions of her mind.

There are other examples of this. Stephen Hawking was diagnosed with motor neuron disease in his early 20s. He survived well past the average 14 months after diagnosis. Stephen went on to become one of the greatest minds in science and contributed immensely to our scientific knowledge. He lived a good life. Perhaps not a perfect life compared with how most of us would measure it, but a good life compared to the one that he had been handed.

What we focus on we get more of. Our mind will give us what it thinks we want. So be really careful what you tell yourself, because you're always listening. What are the things that you're telling yourself? Are they the sorts of things that your best friend would want to hear? If not, you should take note of what it is you're telling yourself. Make sure that it is what you really want.

Now, for a while, I was guilty of this. When I was first diagnosed and not functioning very well, I used to say unhelpful things to myself. Things like, I hate my body, my stupid body – you know, not helpful. It came from frustration and anger. Anger is the first stage of grieving and it's a process that needs to happen. We need to feel the feeling in order to progress. I needed to get to a place where I could accept where I was. Then I could see a way forward as I knew where to start. And if this is you, don't be hard on yourself. A lot of people have the same problem.

Knowing the power of neuroplasticity and its possibilities helped me to shift my focus. Statements became, 'Let's see what I can achieve today and not be too hard on myself,' and 'My body has incredible power to heal itself when I give it what it needs.' By believing in possibility, we override any objections from our subconscious mind. It knows when it's being lied to.

Many of my clients have a problem, and they don't believe it's possible. They do know that they want something different. Their mind has convinced itself that this is how it is. Our mind is partly responsible for this belief. Remember that in keeping us safe it is looking for problems. This is known as a negativity bias. This can make it hard to move past what might seem insurmountable. When something in them says, no, this is not how I want it to be. Let's see what might be possible for me. Shifts can begin to happen.

I once helped a young girl who came to me because the doctors had given up on her. She phoned me up and explained that she'd had two lung transplants and a kidney transplant. She had been told nothing could be done and that she was dying. She had developed a rare infection because she was on immunosuppressant drugs to stop her from rejecting her transplant. Her immune system wasn't able to fight the infection and the treatment for it was damaging her kidney. Her doctors had to stop the treatment. Her lung function was not good and she was struggling to breathe.

We used hypnosis to explore what the core beliefs were about her situation. She was stuck in the memory of rejecting her first transplant. She described the horror of struggling to breathe. This, I felt, was keeping her from getting on top of this infection. I used imagery to help her clear the infection from her body. I helped her to focus her mind on the well person that she had been when she received the second transplant: being the capable young person who had been traveling the world and living life to the full. The mind is so powerful that when she left she was breathing more freely. On top of that, she had some hope restored.

Not everyone wants or needs hypnotherapy in order achieve their goals, but it can definitely help. I used to have lots of people in my classes with all sorts of disabilities. I needed to help them to believe that they could do it. At the very least they needed to believe in the possibility.

I started with what they were telling themselves. I had to ban the word 'can't' in my classes. Before that, I would ask them to try new things, and the response would be, 'no, I can't do that.' We changed it to, 'I'm working towards,' or 'I can, when I learn how, or when I persist,' and other empowering statements like, 'The more I do this, the better I get.' The results were just incredible.

I had people in their mid-80s with post-polio paralysis and Parkinson's disease struggling to get themselves out of bed in the morning, or struggling to stand up from a chair, who, when they really put their minds to it, found that they could. They turned their life around. Faced with being sent to a nursing home, but wanting to remain independent, it was up to them to really put in the work – and they did it. It wasn't me. It was all them just by being really specific with what they wanted.

The same rules apply when we're trying to form new habits. This is especially true around the foods that we eat. Remember, the mind will take us towards something that's pleasurable before something that we don't enjoy or that might cause us pain. So, if you're telling yourself that you can't give up sugar, or can't give up chocolate then your mind won't work for you. But if you tell yourself, 'I'm choosing to eat well' or 'Chocolate and sugar no longer interest me, I choose broccoli,' as long as you're really specific with what you want, your mind will work for you. Simple as that.

So, what do you want? Get really clear because whatever we focus on, we get more of. When we focus on what we can do, the list of what we can do gets bigger. If we focus on what we can't do, well… you know where I'm going with this. What is it that you're going to focus on today? Start with something small, something achievable. Never set yourself up to fail.

Try setting realistic, achievable goals and work towards them little by little. You'll find that a lot of small things start to stack up. And before you know it, you'll look back and wonder how on earth you were ever back there because life is so much better now.

The Seven Stages of Healing

Denial of Problem

Confusion between letting go and unfamiliar 'normal' feelings - cleansing begins.

Anger

Cleansing process begins by blaming others - looking for who/what is responsible - searching for answers.

Bargaining

Guilt and self blame 'should have' - shifting to 'if I do this' - searching for answers.

Depression
Feeling hopeless - grief, pretending you don't care. Letting go - struggle - feeling that no one is listening, including God.

Acceptance
Powerful stage - Accepting responsibility. Procrastination ends - activity begins. Start seeing result of efforts - 'aha!' time. Process speeds up.

Revitalisation
New person in the mirror. Retreat/quiet time - new and delightful discoveries about self. Feeling of empowerment.

Creating a New Life
New opportunities arise. Harmony and peace. Synchronicity. Everything flows with ease. Feeling content.

CHAPTER EIGHT

Stress Less, Live Longer

'Trauma is a fact of life. It does not,
however, have to be a life sentence.'
– Peter A. Levine

It's been long understood and accepted that stress has a big impact on emotional and physical wellbeing. Stress is all around us. It's in our everyday lives. It's on the way to work in busy traffic. It's dealing with the kids whining in the supermarket while you're trying to get through the checkout. It's dealing with that objectionable boss who just doesn't seem to accept that you're doing your best. It's the little trials and tribulations that impact our everyday life. On their own they might not seem like a big deal but they can have a compounding effect.

Stress is a killer and has been implicated in the leading causes of death in our modern society, including things like heart disease, cancer, diabetes, dementia and more. Constant unrelenting stress can cause metabolic dysregulation, leading to inflammation, insulin resistance and a litany of other problems. Our body doesn't know how to deal with it because we are meant to deal with little stresses in the moment and then let them go.

To further explain this, think of a zebra in the African savannah being chased by a lion. That's stressful, and there's only one of two outcomes. Either the zebra gets away or the zebra gets caught and it's over. If the zebra gets away, it stops once it knows it's safe. It shakes off all that stress and just goes back to being a zebra. That's the end of it. It goes back to grazing or whatever it is that zebras do.

Maybe that's how we used to be too. Our society has evolved faster than our physiology has been able to keep up. We have caused ourselves stress and we don't always have healthy methods of dealing with it. Sometimes we turn to unhealthy and destructive behaviours in an attempt to distract ourselves from the unpleasant feelings it creates, like overeating and consuming too much alcohol.

In order to manage everyday unavoidable stress, we can find healthier ways. Taking steps to unwind and have some healthy fun, or spending time doing something we enjoy can at least temporarily give us some relief from our stresses. We can watch a movie, read books, spend time with friends. For some people that can be all they need. For others, they hold onto their stress. It can be related to their BS and the stories that they tell themselves.

On another level, stress can be unrelenting. It's always there. It can feel like you can never get away from it. Like the person who is stuck in an abusive, controlling relationship, or situation who doesn't see that there's any way out. It is often described as feeling like walking on eggshells.

Or the stress of visiting multiple doctors, looking for help but not finding it. Dealing with chronic pain. When there's no escape from that stress, there's also no way for the body to know how to deal with it. So, unrelenting stress has a negative impact on the body.

It might start with a feeling of tension, a strain, sometimes frustration. Muscles might tighten in the neck, in the abdomen and the chest. Heart rate increases and that is a result of the secretion of the hormones, cortisol and adrenaline. Perspiration increases. Our logical thought process can be replaced by irrational and unreasonable thoughts when we're stressed. This is when we make the poorest lifestyle and food choices. This is your amygdala, part of the limbic system, and it takes control to get you out of trouble. It takes priority over the pre-frontal cortex, or thinking brain.

This is why if you are stressed because you are going into an important meeting and you have to perform or because you are going to take a test, you can really struggle to think.

When you have stress, or there is a fear, you are going to have this response where your body at first produces adrenaline then follows up with cortisol. Adrenaline is really quick. It is a neurotransmitter: a quick in and out.

Then cortisol comes in and lasts longer. One of the functions is to increase blood sugar, to fuel up ready to escape. When you're sitting at the desk and the boss is yelling at you, or they have a deadline, or any of the many things that cause stress, cortisol increases your blood sugar. When there is no activity to go with that you don't burn that energy. If there really were a lion chasing you, you would run and get rid of that sugar in the blood. Instead that increased blood sugar goes through the same process as if you had just eaten a meal.

When there is no end to it cortisol causes a rise in inflammation and that can in turn lead to disease.

Some significant life events that may contribute to disease are:

- Death of a spouse
- Divorce
- Separation from a partner
- Detention in gaol or other
- Death of a close family member
- Major personal injury or illness
- Marriage
- Loss of work

Trauma

Trauma can be defined as pretty much anything that causes us to feel overwhelmed. I mentioned ACEs in the last chapter, as they have also been implicated in the development of disease. Further, it can also be physical overwhelm, like heatstroke and exhaustion. It can be traumatic events and accidents. Then we have overwhelming experiences that cause us to be anxious or fearful. So, depending on the level of the stress and how long it continues, it can also become traumatic.

Traumatic experiences can also be stored in the body. This is in addition to the subconscious mind, which is storing it for reference to run it through its filters. The feeling experienced is held as a cellular, or somatic, memory in the body, and can also contribute to disease states.

There have been two interesting areas of research that I'll talk about. The first one is polyvagal theory that was proposed by Dr.

Stephen Porges. His theory examines the vagus nerve. It is the tenth cranial nerve and it connects your brain to your body. It has many branches connecting to all the major organs in your body. It's responsible for communication between the body and the mind and vice versa. It is one of five nerves known collectively as the autonomic nervous system.

It has been long understood that there were two parts to the vagus nerve. The sympathetic and the parasympathetic. The sympathetic nervous system activates our fight or flight response. So, it's primary purpose is to keep you safe. It does that by shutting down all unnecessary functions in the body and redirecting energy so that we can fight or flee. It does so because if we don't manage to survive, well, then all of those functions just became unnecessary.

The parasympathetic nervous system allows the body to rest, digest and repair. Ideally, we need to be in the relaxed parasympathetic for around 90% of our day. When you're asleep and when you're relaxing or just going about your daily business, you should be in a parasympathetic state. That's where everything's functioning well, and there are no undue stresses on body systems. Healing can happen.

Polyvagal Theory

Now, Dr. Porges' theory introduces a new concept, the polyvagal system. He divides the functions of the vagus nerve further. Along with the sympathetic nervous system which is related to threat, he adds the ventral vagal state, where we can relax and engage socially, and bounce back quickly from stressful events. Then there is also shutdown state or dorsal vagal, where we might experience panic attacks, anxiety, obsessive compulsive behaviours and social disconnection. We can get stuck in this state of limbo where we might feel helpless. We can't heal, adequately rest or repair. Unless something changes, we experience chronic disease.

Some feelings and behaviours associated with each state:

Sympathetic/ Threat	Parasympathetic/ Ventral vagal	Dorsal vagal/ Shutdown
Restless	Connected	Exhausted
Hypervigilance	Present	Chronic pain
Anger/Aggression	Grounded	Depression
Insomnia	Healthy	Overwhelm
Teeth grinding	Calm	Disconnection

Cell Danger Response

The second is the theory of the cell danger response, by Robert Niavaux, MD, PhD. He theorises that there is also a metabolic response that is happening at the cellular level. It involves the mitochondria. There are millions of them and they are responsible for producing cellular energy. That's their primary function, but their secondary function is as part of the immune and/or danger response.

Their function when they sense danger is to shut down energy production. If you're being invaded by some nasty pathogen, say a virus or bacteria, it will attempt to harness your mitochondria for energy. They will then use that energy to replicate and invade the body. So, it's a protective mechanism.

Niavaux proposes that chronic disease is a consequence of the healing cycle being blocked. The response fails to turn back off. The cells basically get caught in a never-ending loop, unable to completely recover. In other words, chronic disease is caused by a biological reaction to an injury.

We can get stuck in the cell danger response and also in dorsal vagal. Both of these theories tie in with well with the hypothesis of infections triggering autoimmunity. They also add weight to traumatic experiences contributing to chronic disease states.

A lot of functional medicine practitioners also believe that all illness begins in the gut, which as we know is connected to the vagus. The theory also offers an explanation as to how sufferers of chronic fatigue syndrome struggle to function, lacking the energy to even get out of bed. It is as though something has shut off energy production.

So, what can we do about it? Well, we can look at the sorts of stresses and traumas that have happened in our lives and try to make sense of them. We can look at our experiences through a new lens. If X happened to me when I was seven years old and it's still potentially impacting me now that I'm in my adulthood, is it still relevant? Can I teach my mind and/or body that it no longer needs to be responding in this way? Is the meaning that I attached to that event still true?

Now, an example of this might be from back when I was a seven-year-old. We were impacted by bush fires. I remember the colour of the sky and not much else. Beyond that I only know from the stories that my parents shared with me. I don't remember being particularly fearful, although I'm sure that my parents' response would have added a sense of what was happening.

My mind and body remembered though. I became very sensitive to the smell of smoke and would develop a sense of unease whenever I saw a bushfire sun. There's a particular look about the sky or something that triggers that memory. I have often known there were nearby fires before I could see or smell smoke.

That experience would have been soaked up by my nervous system. My subconscious mind made its own judgement call. Our sense of smell is very important for our safety. It can tell us if food is safe to eat, or alert us to danger when we smell gas or smoke.

But what about if you don't actually remember any traumas? You might not even be aware of them. They could have happened when you were too young to even know that they happened. It could have been something as simple as your mother experienced some postnatal depression, and she wasn't really available for you. Or, like my mother, she could have been busy with the demands of her own unwell mother. I don't know it as fact, but it's possible that I didn't get my needs met at times when I was a baby.

Or the client that I had who was diagnosed with fibromyalgia. It's a complex pain syndrome that is not well understood and often dismissed by doctors as not a 'real' disorder. Utilising hypnosis we examined the time that she had been beaten as a young child for something that wasn't her fault. Not only was there the physical trauma of the abuse, but also the shame, humiliation and sense of injustice that the 'responsible' adult present had failed to prevent it.

The pain was there as a reminder to avoid similar situations. A simple visit with family would make her ten times worse, leading to avoidance of family gatherings. It was causing disharmony in her marriage and distress over lost enjoyment of activities.

Understanding that the pain was recurring to protect her was liberating. We needed to work on establishing a sense of safety and control in order for her to get better.

Anything is possible and we won't necessarily know. What we can know is how we feel in certain situations, such as noticing that every time something happens we get a headache or stomach ache – whatever it might be for you. We first need to acknowledge what we feel. It's there for a reason and sometimes we need to feel it until it no longer needs to be felt.

We do so by reminding ourselves that we are safe. No matter what happened when I was a child, I'm no longer a child. I'm a responsible adult, responsible for my own destiny. Allowing ourselves to express how we feel is important even if we can only tell the cat, or the wall. Write it down, keep a journal. Find what works for you and seek help if you need it.

We can learn to move our nervous system into the parasympathetic state. Simply by breathing in slowly through your nose for a count of four, holding it and then breathing out slowly we can move towards parasympathetic. Humming your favourite tune or vigorously gargling will do the same. A lot of people recommend keeping a gratitude journal. If that's not your thing, simply think of something that you appreciate. Imagine relaxing in your favourite place: hear the sounds, feel the breeze or warmth of the sun.

We have the power to use our minds to imagine anything. So, see yourself in a place of safety. Notice that feeling in your body that first raises the alarm; you'll know it if you have it. It's often in the stomach or chest area. You can instruct your body to let it go. There are a number of things that can help if that doesn't work. I use a range of techniques like tapping, somatic experiencing and visualisation. Once you change the meaning of events and release stored traumas from the body, you can begin to heal.

There are lots of ways to mitigate stress. Find something that works for you. Try walks in nature. Take your shoes off and feel the grass or sand, play with the kids. Laugh and have fun. Find a way to let it go. If it's the drive to work instead of bemoaning the traffic, turn it around, flip it on its head: I'm so lucky to have this time to be able to listen to my favourite podcast on the way to work or enjoy my favourite music. Take the time sitting at the lights to be working through a to-do list for tomorrow or plan a picnic with friends. You can reframe unavoidable tasks into something that is no longer stressful. Your body will thank you.

CHAPTER NINE

Get Your Sleep Together

'There is a time for many words,
and there is also a time for sleep.'
– Homer, The Odyssey

I cannot overstate the importance of sleep. We can tend to think it's okay to miss sleep, thinking, 'I'll sleep tomorrow or catch up on the weekend.' The fact is we all need seven to nine hours of quality sleep every night. We need sleep for a number of good reasons. So, what is happening when we sleep?

It is known that as we sleep, we cycle through four phases. The first is where we start to lose conscious awareness, or 'fall asleep.' Once asleep, we have a period of light sleep, which is similar to a short nap. It can last for about 20 minutes. In both of these stages it can feel as though you are awake even though you are not. Then we move into the deep sleep stage, which can last around an hour where we will be much harder to wake.

Finally, we move into REM or rapid eye movement, where we do most of our dreaming. During this stage you become mostly paralysed and it's thought that is to prevent us from hurting ourselves if we have a bad dream. In this stage, the brain is as active as if we were awake and moving around. The eyes are moving in a rapid motion as if watching something, but no one really knows why. We continue to cycle through these stages as many as four or five times in a night.

So, what else is the body doing while you sleep, you might wonder? Remember the parasympathetic state that we talked about in chapter eight? Well, ideally you're in that state while you sleep. Let's start from the top and work our way down.

Number one, sleep washes our brain. Yes, you read that right, washes. A relatively new discovery is the glymphatic system. While you're in deep sleep, your brain pulsates. That might sound a little unbelievable but it has been studied. It does this because there actually isn't a circulatory system in the brain. So, what happens is it pulsates and forces cerebrospinal fluid (CSF) through the tissues. CSF surrounds the brain providing nourishment and protection.

As you sleep it washes through your brain removing any toxins or dead and damaged cells. This shows how important sleep is especially as we age and it naturally becomes lighter. We also need to remove other waste including toxic proteins like tau and beta amyloid that have been associated with Alzheimer's.

Besides cleaning house, we're sorting through all of our learnings, and filing away memories. The brain is busy deciding what needs to be kept and what can be pruned. This is neuroplasticity at work. The more a neural pathway is in use the stronger it becomes, while seldom or never used pathways are downgraded.

Your body also has a lot of work to do while you sleep. It's producing new cells. It's also taking the cells that are damaged or past their use by date and recycling them. It's taking the proteins that it can, breaking them down and reusing them to build new cells. The liver is busy detoxifying and it's also burning fat as fuel. Sleep is also vital for your hormones to be in balance.

Remember that when we're under stress, our cortisol rises. It also has another important job. And that is to wake you up in the morning. So, in an ideal world, your cortisol levels are at their peak in the morning to wake you up. Providing you're in parasympathetic mode, as you should be for the rest of your day, then your cortisol levels will drop right down. So that by the time you want to go to sleep, they're at their lowest. And then as they're dropping your melatonin is kicking in to help you to sleep.

Growth hormone and DHEA rise, to help with cellular repair and to stimulate the growth of new cells, including brain cells. DHEA is like the master hormone: it's converted to adrenaline, cortisol, oestrogen, progesterone and testosterone. Progesterone is produced by men too and it also assists with restful sleep.

And while we're on the subject of hormones, you have another hormone that rises and falls in opposition to cortisol. That's leptin. So, while cortisol is high in the morning, your leptin should be low. Then during the day, it starts to rise. Leptin is a signalling hormone that's produced by your fat cells. It tells you when you've had enough to eat. It has to reach its peak then fall to allow growth hormone to rise while you sleep.

What happens if you don't get enough sleep? Well, it all gets muddled up. If you're tired, you'll be more inclined to want to eat more. As insulin sensitivity decreases, it causes you to eat more as glucose can't get into your cells. So you produce more insulin, dropping your blood sugar and you'll then have a rise in your cortisol, which then raises your insulin dropping your blood sugar and making you hungry.

You can see where I'm going with this: it all starts to get out of kilter. Just one night of poor sleep will temporarily throw off the balance. Consistently getting poor sleep is setting you up for disease. Consistently higher insulin makes the cells resistant. This is the beginning of diabetes if nothing changes. When leptin is out of balance we can lose sensitivity to it as well, making it difficult to maintain a healthy weight.

Some tips to getting a good night's sleep. Don't eat for at least three hours before bedtime. There's a couple of reasons for that. First, if you eat too close to bedtime, you won't get the rise in melatonin because insulin will prevent it, making it hard to get restorative sleep. Secondly, Leptin will peak too late preventing the spike in growth hormone, which means you won't get all those benefits of new cellular growth and repair happening overnight, including fat loss, because you'll miss your peak.

Let's talk more about melatonin. It's produced by your pineal gland and it is affected by light. Studies have shown that even people with total blindness have melatonin levels reduced by light exposure. Melatonin production is turned on by low light. It is also protective against tumour growth, in particular breast cancer.

This is why it's important to turn off your screen at least one or two hours before bed. Screens emit blue light, which is naturally present in sunlight and supposed to be at its highest during daytime. We can use a filter on our phone or computer but it's really hard to put a filter on your TV. So, if you're up late watching TV you're being exposed to a lot blue light.

If you can, turn off the TV at least an hour before you plan to go to bed and give your melatonin a chance to kick in. Dim the lights in your home because the artificial light that we use alters our circadian rhythm. Unlike our ancestors who lived in caves, and had to rely on fire for light. They naturally slept when the sun set and rose at dawn. We need to emulate that as best we can.

It's also important to look at gut health. If you have problems with your digestion, you may not be producing neurotransmitters efficiently like serotonin. It's important for mental health but it is also a precursor to melatonin. In order to produce enough you need good nutrition. Addressing food sensitivities is another overlooked area. High histamine from foods can act as an excitatory neurotransmitter, meaning it wakes you up. Alcohol is just one example of a histamine 'food'.

When we retire for the night, we really want to be in a nice dark room. Adding extra window coverings can help if you have light pollution from street lighting or neighbouring buildings. Even if you wear a sleep mask there are light receptors in the skin, so darken the room if you can. Add an extra set of curtains. I have even seen shift workers cover their windows in aluminium foil in order to optimise sleep during the day.

Our bodies like to be a bit cooler when we sleep. Use a fan if you have to. If you're in an air-conditioned home, set the thermostat at no more than 19 degrees Celsius overnight, because if you're too warm, you just won't get a good quality sleep. Even during the cooler months, you should avoid using too many blankets.

Find ways to wind down before sleep that will help you relax. Meditation and visualisations before bed can turn down cortisol. If you have something on your mind, keep a journal by the bed and write it down. Getting it out of your head will help you to wind down.

Think of three things you appreciated today. Taking a warm bath works for some people but not all so see what works best for you. Lavender essential oil can be added to the bath or use a diffuser if you like the scent. Try a cup of chamomile or lemon balm tea, as both are said to help relax the body and mind.

One thing that I like to do is to monitor my sleep. For that I use a Fitbit. Now there are a few companies that produce similar devices. I have tried a couple but I've found this to be best for me. It monitors my sleep, giving a good indication of how well I slept the night before. I can see a trend and troubleshoot problems in real time.

It also gives me other information that I find useful, like my activity level. Getting enough movement in the day also helps with sleep. Make sure to get some exercise during the day, but not too close to bedtime. A little intense movement for a couple of minutes, perhaps an hour or two before you intend to go to bed, is okay. It can help to stimulate your growth hormone.

The Fitbit also shows me other health metrics that my inner geek loves, like heart rate variability. It's another way to monitor parasympathetic activation. That in turn alerts me to take steps to identify and manage any additional stress.

I can identify in real-time things that are impacting my sleep. Obviously, if I drink too much coffee during the day, I'm not going to sleep as well. That's a no-brainer. But if I have one glass of wine with my dinner, I'm okay, interestingly enough. More than that and I won't sleep as well. Bottom line, it's not good for my sleep. Another good reason for keeping a journal.

If you think that you not getting quality sleep, despite addressing the aforementioned, you can ask your doctor for a referral for a sleep study. Has anyone told you that you snore? You could be experiencing sleep apnoea. This is a condition where breathing is obstructed leading to disruptions in sleep. Untreated, it is exposing you to a higher risk of adverse health implications like stroke, type 2 diabetes and even dementia.

If you're not sleeping well, you really need to draw your attention to it. Create a sleep routine that you follow and practice good sleep hygiene. It can be really hard to learn to quiet that brain down so that we can go to sleep. The good news is there are ways to train your brain to slow down. You can download a relaxation recording from my website.

Some tips for sound sleep

- Get some morning sun as soon as you can once you wake up
- Plan to be in bed no later than 10 pm
- Sleep in as dark an environment as possible
- Manage your stress
- Stop eating three hours before bedtime
- Turn off or dim lights after sunset
- Have a bedtime ritual

CHAPTER TEN

You Are What You Eat

'You are what you eat. So don't be fast, cheap, easy, or fake.'

You may well think that you have heard it all before. There have been a lot of celebrities, doctors and dieticians out there that have come up with diets. I've even followed some myself, but they don't suit everyone. Some of them are simply dangerous, like the fresh air diet. One poor woman met her death by following that one.

Some are hopelessly outdated and offer advice that has been found to be counterproductive. Or they can be so restrictive that they can be difficult to stick with and even nutritionally devoid. When it comes to diet, there is no one-size-fits-all. There are sound guidelines, but individuality determines what is best for each of us.

There are a few basic guidelines that you should pay attention to. Number one is to drink plenty of water, but preferably not straight from the tap. It can contain chemicals from the treatment process and other impurities. If you can drink it filtered that is better. You can get an under-sink system installed at reasonable cost. Even ceramic countertop systems remove impurities and improve the quality. You can even buy purified water if filtering the tap water is not enough or not possible.

On that note, ideally do not drink out of a plastic bottle. Water should not be stored in plastic either. There are lots of stainless steel and glass drink bottles available these days. Swap the plastic and do yourself, and the environment, a favour.

Our bodies are on average made up of 60% water. Guidelines have long been to drink between six and eight glasses of water a day. That fails to take into account the water contained in foods and beverages that we consume. It also doesn't allow for environmental variations like sweating more in hot weather.

I find a better indicator is the colour of your pee. It should be pale yellow like straw when you're fully hydrated. If you're thirsty, you are already somewhat dehydrated. Interestingly thirst sometimes triggers hunger so drink a glass of water first especially if it hasn't been long since you last ate. And speaking of pee, it's your kidneys flushing out waste. If you don't drink enough you make their job harder. Conversely drinking too much makes them work harder to maintain fluid and electrolyte balance.

Fast

Coming back to the quote at the beginning of this chapter, don't be fast. Here, fast refers to fast food. It's not really the best; it's just convenient. It's okay in moderation, but just don't do it every day. Ideally, don't do it more than once a year. I will only consider it if there's nothing else available and I get caught short, like if I'm traveling. Even then, I skip the fries and sugary drinks that come with it. Choose wisely.

Cheap

If it's cheap, you often get what you pay for, like the student staple two-minute noodles. Its nutritional value can be very questionable: high in salt, artificial flavours and often saturated fat. Uggh! Choose the best food that you can afford. Aim for fresh food and organic, if you can. Vegetables should account for ideally 80% of what we eat. Sorry, chips don't count as vegetables.

Easy

Now for easy. Well, there's a lot of easy options out there to think of. The freezer section of your supermarket is packed with them: just 'bung it in the microwave and heat it up' meals. While they might be easy, and they're often marketed as healthy, they are mass-produced and not necessarily the best choice.

Then there's the canned and packaged off-the-shelf ready-to-go meals. I don't know about you but a chicken meal that doesn't require refrigeration and has a use by date a year from now... are you really getting the best quality nutrients from foods when they're presented in that way?

Would you be better off skipping that aisle and cooking from scratch? There's plenty of choice in the fresh food aisles. It doesn't have to be too complicated. There's lots of recipes and cooking demonstrations available online. There are also good recipe books offering easy to put together, fresh and healthy meals.

Fake

And that brings us to fake. I often refer to it as 'Franken-food.' This has become an interesting topic lately. I've seen a lot of meat-free 'meat' products, like no-meat pizzas and no-meat pies. These things that are promoted as being vegetarian or vegan. But they're fake food. They're not real food and they're highly processed.

They might be processed from vegetable matter, but are they anything like the vegetables that they started with? And do you really need something that looks and possibly tastes like a meat pie anyway? When it comes to food, you want it to be nourishing and sustaining, not novelty.

And then, I would add to that, if you can't or couldn't make it at home in your own kitchen, then why would you be eating it now? And I'm not talking about the stuff that the gourmet chefs produce. I'm talking about things like candy, gummy lollies, potato chips. There are kids snacks marketed as healthy because they're made from fruit. You are winding up with a bunch of artificial additives, sweeteners, colourings and flavours.

Would your grandmother recognise it as food? Can you recreate those in your kitchen? If you couldn't even begin to know where to start, then please really consider whether or not you should be eating it.

Make no mistake: the food manufacturers want you to keep coming back. In fact, I had a client once, back when I was a personal trainer, who came to me for assistance with weight loss. She was a grossly overweight lady. A lovely person, who worked as a professional food taster for one of the big companies that produced frozen, ready-to-go meals. And her size said it all. She would spend all day tasting that food. She was employed to make it taste better so people want to come back and buy more of it. And it was not doing her any good at all.

When I asked her, she said, 'Well, yeah, it's all about the taste. We have to put things in there that we know people like. People like salty. People like sweet. People like tasty, whatever it is that people keep coming back for. We keep adding it to the food and make sure they buy more of it.' It's the same with fast food like KFC's 11 secret herbs and spices. Well, the secret is that they're putting them there to make you keep coming back for more. That's it! Bottom line: it empties your wallet and feeds your waistline. Your health may suffer but the company profits.

Eat well

So how do we get down to the nitty-gritty of what we should eat? There is so much information. Go paleo, ketogenic, autoimmune paleo, south beach, low fat, no sugar, fruitarian. Do this, don't do that. It's overwhelming, so we give up and go back to old habits. I prefer the KISS principle. Keep it simple…

The Mediterranean diet is a good starting point that can be modified fairly easily to exclude certain foods if required. We need a modest amount of good quality protein: 1-1.5 mg per kilogram of bodyweight per day for the average adult. That's around the size of the palm of your hand if you're eating animal protein.

Aim to eat the rainbow every day. Include a variety of vegetables but focus mainly on non-starchy and green leafy vegetables. Including some nuts, seeds and beans will provide extra protein as well as healthy fats and fibre. Add a couple of serves of low glycaemic fruit. Berries are packed with antioxidants and are a good choice.

Digestion matters

Make sure that you're eating the best quality that you can. Sit down to eat, take your time – it shouldn't be a rush. Chew your food. It seems obvious but we can get in the habit of shovelling it in. Digestion starts in your mouth. Amylase, an enzyme in saliva, starts to break down starches. This triggers the release of hydrochloric acid in the stomach.

The stomach is a highly acidic environment. This serves as a safety mechanism against food-borne bacteria and other pathogens. It also helps to digest the food further. As it passes further down into the small intestine, the liver sends bile via the gallbladder to help digest fats. The pancreas adds in enzymes to help with the further breakdown of proteins and carbohydrates. You need all of these to happen in order to absorb the nutrients from your food.

While we're talking digestion there seems to be a lot of waste involved. Yes, I'm talking poop. It's worth paying attention to as well. Ideally, we are pooping at least once a day. Your liver is busy detoxing your blood and breaking down any medications or toxins from your environment. It is recycling the old cells that I mentioned in chapter nine. It sends anything water soluble to the kidneys but everything else goes out via poop. You don't want it hanging around for too long as your colon, or large intestine, will reabsorb toxins along with water. Then the liver has to do it all again.

This wouldn't be complete without mentioning the other function of our colon. It houses billions and billions of bacteria and other microorganisms, known as the microbiome. Their job is to further breakdown anything that hasn't yet been digested. They extract B vitamins which are reabsorbed to be used in many essential processes like producing our neurotransmitters.

Microbes also produce vitamin K so that our blood can clot to repair damage and essential fatty acids to keep cell membranes healthy. They love fibre: it's their favourite food. It also keeps things moving along and sweeps the surface, clearing away old cells and other debris.

The microbiome is as individual as you are. The microorganisms have been affected over time by many things, in particular antibiotics. Nearly everyone has been treated with them and they can alter the make-up of the microbiome. Some of our bacteria serve to neutralise harmful substances in food, like the oxalates found in foods like spinach. Plants use them as protection against chewing insects.

If not broken down, they can form sharp crystals that can migrate anywhere in the body and cause havoc. That, in turn, raises inflammation. They also can rob the body of minerals, like calcium and magnesium. Oxalates tend to bind with them, making them unavailable. They can be found in a lot of foods substituted for gluten. Be careful of nut flours in particular as they are very high in oxalates. You can't accurately test for them which is why paying attention to symptoms over time is so valuable.

Give yourself an oil change

Next, I would suggest that we all need an oil change. Just as your car needs good clean oil, so do you. You may have been consuming vegetable oils. Polyunsaturated oils like sunflower and canola are not what we need. These can be altered by heat which makes them more like saturated fat and are highly processed. They are too high in omega six oils that increase inflammation. Ideally, choose extra-virgin cold pressed olive oil to drizzle over salads. For cooking, if you must, use a little extra virgin coconut oil.

We also need omega 3 oils for DHA and EPA from fish, or a good quality supplement. They are anti-inflammatory and help to keep the membranes of our cells nice and flexible. You need a 20:1 balance of omega 3 to omega 6. While there are plant sources of alpha lineolic acid, like flaxseed, the bodies capacity to convert it to DHA is very low and not enough to solely rely on.

Your brain needs more fat to maintain myelin, the insulating coating on our nerves, than the rest of you, so make sure it's the good stuff. Beyond that, there's not many oils that I would recommend. We just don't need them. We don't need too much either, just a Goldilocks amount – around 10-15% of your daily calorie intake. There's nine calories in every gram of fat, so that's around two tablespoons a day.

Food intolerance

We should pay attention to how food affects us. I can't tell you how many times I've had people say to me, 'Well, when I eat too much bread I get bloated. Or if I have toast in the morning, but then I have pasta at night, then I get bloated. Worse still if I eat X then I will spend hours on the toilet.' Well, your body's trying to tell you something. And it's probably telling you that you've got a sensitivity to either wheat or gluten. Gluten is said to be a problem for everyone.

This came about through the findings of some scientific research that I read a few years ago. It found that every single one of us, when we eat gluten, in order to digest it, it stimulates the release of an enzyme called zonulin. And what it does is it actually opens up the gaps between cells known as tight junctions.

The gut is lined with a single layer of cells, called endothelial cells. It's designed like netting or a fine sieve and its purpose is to be just large enough to allow good food particles through and into the bloodstream. So, as we digest our food it can be transported to the cells, while keeping all the other things out. But what zonulin does is loosen up the gaps between the cells, which starts to make little holes in our net that we may not be able to heal.

Over time, the holes can get bigger and allow foreign things through. That's where the term 'leaky gut' comes from. Some of us are perhaps more susceptible to it, but certainly over time, it can cause really big problems. It also raises inflammation as the immune system senses that there is damage occurring.

One of the problems is that when our gut is leaking, the wrong particles or proteins are coming through into our bloodstream and our immune systems are alerted. It's like, 'Wait a minute, what's this thing it's not supposed to be here? I don't recognise it, but I'll take note of it.' Then over time it starts a process called molecular mimicry that might be triggered by an infection or inflammation.

It becomes a problem when the substance that came through our gut starts to look a little bit like, say, the myelin on our nerves. Perhaps it looks a little bit like the cartilage in our joints. Or it looks a little bit like any cell you can imagine. There are over 80 autoimmune conditions documented. So that can be a problem. Wouldn't you agree? Taking note of how food's affecting us is very important. Do consider whether you really need to be consuming gluten at all.

In addition, while we're still on the topic of leaky endothelial cells, all of our blood vessels are lined with endothelial cells. If you stretched out all of yours, they could circle the earth just over two times. I don't know about you but I don't want to risk leakage. The blood-brain barrier is the most well known as it protects the organ that's running the show. Food for thought, if you'll pardon the pun.

Food sensitivities are quite different to food allergies. Allergies are fairly obvious. And if you have an allergy, you'll usually know about it; from sneezing and itching due to hives or rashes, or, at the extreme end of the scale your lips can swell or you might have trouble breathing. At its worst, you can have what's known as an anaphylactic reaction. It's life-threatening. That's one of the common things that we see in people with peanut allergies, for example.

Gluten intolerance is well known due to its implications in celiac disease. However, you can become sensitive to pretty much anything. Sensitivities can come and go depending on the state of your overall wellbeing. Somebody can be reacting to a substance in a food today, but over time that can be improved. Or it could be that they are intolerant and will need to avoid it for rest of their life. These are not taken as seriously as life-threatening allergies, and there's no way to really test accurately for them.

The best way to know is by first taking note of any symptoms you have. They can be subtle. It can be things like changes in your mood. I have a nephew that would behave aggressively whenever he ate avocado. The most problematic foods tend to be gluten, dairy, eggs, corn and soy.

There are many substances in foods like salicylates, oxalates, phenols and amines that can also be problematic. You do need to pay attention over time, because you might not see a reaction to a food for up to three days. It could be that something that you ate on Monday is making you feel sad and miserable and just all out of sorts on Thursday. Or it can be as simple as yesterday I ate pumpkin, today I've got a headache.

You won't know unless you pay attention over a period of time and track it backwards and look for the patterns. I use known signs and symptoms to help me to identify likely foods but that is beyond the scope of this chapter. Once you think you have identified the culprit/s they need to be eliminated from your diet for some time to be sure. Give it a couple of weeks at least before testing to see if it's still a problem. It's trial and error and can change over time.

Sugar matters

And, of course, the big one: you need to keep your blood sugar in balance. That means not eating too many starchy carbohydrates that spike your blood sugar and raise your insulin. Aim more for whole grains and whole foods. Things with a bit of fibre in them give you a much better, slower release of the energy from your food. They won't cause your insulin to spike, and you won't get the drop in your blood sugar that follows.

Having balanced blood sugar gives your body a more constant source of energy. When it's in balance it's not stressed either. You don't want excess sugar running around in your blood stream, as it's really damaging. If your blood sugar is not in balance you can become insulin resistant. Your cells are screaming for energy, but the insulin receptors become damaged and they don't function as well. So, the body keeps pumping out more insulin, and you are constantly tired and hungry. Now you've become insulin resistant. It's going to be causing a lot of damage to your body.

High blood sugar has been shown to be a big problem in heart disease, possibly more so than cholesterol, as it raises inflammation in the body. That sets off a cascade of problems. Your doctor might put you on medication to help your body produce more insulin. Over time that can damage your pancreas and it gives up. Then you might require insulin injections.

Besides heart disease, uncontrolled high blood sugar damages nerves. Alzheimer's disease has been dubbed 'type 3 diabetes' by some in the medical community as high levels of insulin are extremely damaging to sensitive brain cells. It can cause eye problems like cataracts and eventually blindness. It damages the blood vessels and can cause peripheral vascular disease leading to potential amputation. It can also cause kidney failure. Now if any of that scares you – and it should – the good news is it can be reversed. In most cases it can, unless the damage to the pancreas, and other organs, is too great.

Bottom line

At the end of the day, what this all means is to eat the best quality food you can. Food can harm or food can heal. Pay attention to any changes in your body or mood. Remember the vagus nerve? The gut is often referred to as the second brain. It's communicating with the brain giving constant feedback on the state of play. If you have inflammation in the gut, it's impacting the whole body.

CHAPTER ELEVEN

Use It or Lose It

'What we need is to use what we have.'
– Susan Sontag

Our bodies were designed to move, but our modern life has us sitting down way too much. We spend so much time in a chair, behind a desk, on the phone or keyboard. I would argue that it's getting worse, particularly at the moment in the middle of this current pandemic. We had been heading this way for too long already. Now many of us are working from home, we don't even have to get up and walk out the door.

We used to walk to the bus stop or get in the car and drive to the city, park and then walk from the parking station to the office. Now if we want, we can fall out of bed and throw on a track suit. Maybe we only need to get half-dressed to be properly attired for a video meeting. We can stumble from the bedroom to the kitchen and then to the office, wherever that may be in our home, spend time at the desk and then rinse and repeat.

Without our colleagues to go and have lunch with, for example, we can just spend all of our time in the house. It's much, much harder to motivate ourselves to move. But movement's really important for our body. It keeps our detox systems working.

Now we talked about the glymphatic system in the brain. Well, it links into the lymphatic system, which is a third circulatory system that's running throughout the body. It doesn't have a pump or anything else to move it around. In the same way that the brain has to pulsate to move its glymphatic system, your muscles need to move to pump your lymphatic system. It's particularly important for the lower limbs, because they're working against the most gravity.

Next, we need to move to keep our joints healthy. Movement stimulates the lining inside each joint to release synovial fluid. It nourishes and lubricates the cartilage lining the bones to limit wear and tear. Even if you already have some arthritis, it's still vital to move. Freeing up creaky joints will improve pain, and help to limit further damage.

It's not only gravity and weight-bearing that maintain bone density. Movement keeps our bones strong. Muscle tugs on bone stimulating it to utilise calcium and build strong bone cells. It's ideal to add weight-bearing exercise to your daily routine. Walking is a great addition if you can. Incorporating some strength training is vital to avoid osteoporosis. It's not something I would wish on anyone. I once had a client who had suffered multiple fractures. It was so bad that she could break a rib by simply sneezing.

A side benefit is that you build more muscle. That helps with everyday activities. Making mundane things like carrying the groceries more like a walk in the park. You also need enough muscle that you can regain your balance to prevent falls. If you're able to get up on your feet at all, then you should. You need to be safely challenging your balance. It's vitally important as statistics show that if you fall and break a hip, there's a very good chance that you will not return to the same life that you had.

Your body likes to conserve energy. It does this by only utilising what it needs to. When it comes to muscles, if you don't use them, your body will turn them off. Muscle fibres get put into retirement because it takes energy to maintain them. If you're not using them, why waste precious resources?

The same goes for those energy-producing cells that I mentioned in chapter eight. If you're not utilising mitochondria, they will also be downsized, both in size and number. So, if you're not utilising your muscles – which by the way, contain the most mitochondria – they'll also turn off and you wind up less able. You might remember spending time in bed with the flu, or an injury. Your mitochondria would have been reduced and shut down. You likely would have felt like you had decreased energy until they built up again as you recovered.

Now, couple that with the fact that we lose mitochondria anyway, naturally as we age. As we age, we also lose the capacity to build and retain muscle, and it begins in our 40s. That means it's even more important to keep using it because if you don't, well, of course, you're going to lose it. We want to maintain what we have ideally, and even build up some more. Yes, building up more is possible, even as we age.

It's obvious that movement burns energy. The side benefit is that it also reduces triglycerides and helps to manage your cholesterol. That in turn helps to lower the inflammation in your body. Muscle also has greater insulin sensitivity, which means that your muscles are able to take up glucose more efficiently and burn it as energy, so you don't wind up with as many cells that are resistant to blood sugar. You use up glucose so that it's not floating around causing problems in your blood vessels.

When your blood vessels are not inflamed, they're nice and flexible as they should be, which helps to maintain normal blood pressure. When your blood vessels are rigid and inflexible, then your blood pressure will be raised. It's a little bit like trying to water the garden with a kink in the hose: the pressure builds up. This, in turn, puts you at greater risk of cardiovascular disease, heart attack, stroke and more.

Anything is better than nothing. It doesn't have to be in a gym, just do what you can. I've had many clients over the years that couldn't get out of a chair. Some of them were in a wheelchair. For my classes held in retirement homes, many were barely able to shuffle to a chair from their room. We were still able to do some effective exercise in a chair.

You don't even need to use weights. You can improvise and use household items. A one kilo bag of rice can double as a weight and can even be tied to a limb with a sock or scarf. Empty milk bottles filled with water or a can of baked beans can also work. Start somewhere, be consistent and you will soon find that you can manage more.

Easy, simple exercises can be found online as well. A side benefit of the pandemic is that there are many free YouTube videos to choose from. Make sure to clear it with you doctor and use common sense to pick something suitable for your situation. If you can find yourself a good personal trainer or exercise physiologist, even better.

If you have physical mobility issues or other limitations, you need somebody who can really be on board. They can modify exercises so that they are suitable for you. It's even possible to do modified yoga in a chair. Pilates was developed during the first world war by Joseph Pilates in order to help rehabilitate injured soldiers in their beds!

If you're able to get out and about, a walk in nature does absolute wonders for lowering stress and improving your mental wellbeing. In fact, Japanese forest bathing, or *shinrin yoku* has been shown in studies to reduce both cortisol and blood pressure. If you can, take your shoes off and feel your feet on the ground. Walking on the beach and breathing in the salt air, feeling the sun on your skin are all positive steps towards better health.

I love dance as exercise. I also used to incorporate some dance into my classes. We had fun, but that's what it's all about. Have some fun, get some movement. Most of all, pick something fun. If you enjoy something you will do it consistently. Remember we like things that are pleasurable more than painful. Your mind believes what you tell it so make it enjoyable. If for some reason you can't get out there and move, turn the music up and dance like nobody's watching.

On the topic of classes: attending a regular class does more than improve your health through increased fitness. In chapter seven, I mentioned safety. Dating back to prehistoric times, being a part of a tribe was crucial to survival. Getting to know your fellow classmates satisfies this primal need. We are social beings. Spending time with others makes us feel safe as we develop a sense of connection and belonging. This is even more important as we age and retire from work.

Water is a fabulous medium for exercising. If you can, swimming is really good for you. It improves cardiovascular fitness. But if you can't swim, just walking in water is really beneficial. Water is a very supportive environment. It reduces the effect of gravity and can take up to 70% of the load off the joints compared to land. The downside is that is harder to use it to increase bone density, but it's not impossible.

Water is actually seven times more resistant than air. So, you're getting seven times the bang for your buck in terms of strengthening your muscles, just by pushing through the water. There are aqua fitness classes that are available in pools around the world. They cater for different levels of fitness and ability. There are even lanes set aside for walking at some public pools.

Pools can be indoors, outdoors, cold or warm water. So, make sure you find one that's suitable to your level of capability. Some will require that you get medical clearance from your doctor. Do check with your doctor because the extra pressure of water slightly increases the strain on your heart until you get used to the environment and adapt.

I should mention HIIT or high intensity interval training. It's one of the latest exercise styles that is being promoted by fitness professionals and some functional medicine practitioners. It has shown many benefits. The premise is that you go hard, say run for a minute, then walk for two. This pattern is repeated for 15 minutes, or more. It is thought to achieve better results for time spent than more traditional exercise.

Even 30 seconds of higher intensity movement has been shown to increase BDNF. What's that? Brain derived neurotropic factor. In plain English, it stimulates the growth of new brain cells. It can be anything that raises you heart rate. Even rapidly punching the air will do it. We don't always need vigorous exercise. It could be something to work towards but any movement is better than no movement. After all, if you don't move it, you really are going to lose it. Most of all, be safe and make it fun.

CHAPTER TWELVE

Solving the Puzzle

———— • ————

*'You may never know what results come of your actions, but if
you do nothing, there will be no results.'*
– Mahatma Gandhi

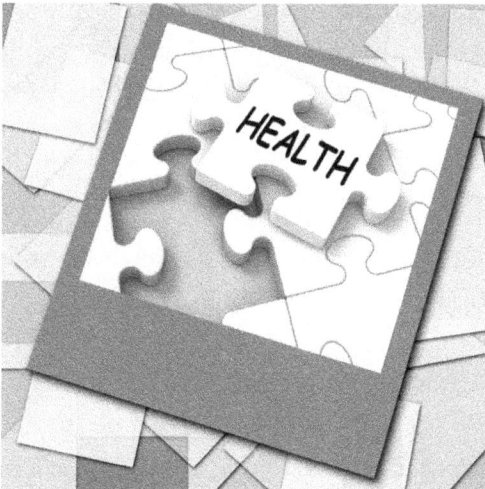

Congratulations on reading this far. I know that it can be a lot to take in. I might have introduced some new ideas compared to what you may have been led to believe. So now for your next steps.

Your challenge, if you choose to accept it, is to just start somewhere. Be curious about what you can learn about your body. Remember we all have a different experience of even the same event. Resist comparing your progress to others. Measure any changes against yourself.

Only then will you begin to shift your beliefs and perspective about disease. Remember the label that have may have been applied to you is just a diagnostic tool. You don't own it and there's no need to wear it. Your doctor has done his or her best to apply their best knowledge and treat you accordingly. They don't live in your body. You do. They don't know all of your experiences. You do.

That does not mean you should not continue to work with them. You do need to feel comfortable with them. Trust is important, as is good communication. In fact, the best partnership with your doctor is one where you feel free to ask questions. It's equally important to receive an explanation that you understand. You need to be involved in any decisions.

If you need to find a new doctor for any reason, start by doing some research. Ask for local referrals or reviews. You can often find them online these days. Go to your appointments well prepared. Take any relevant reports or referrals with you. Make a list of any questions that you want to ask and take notes so that you can refer back to them. At the appointment, did the doctor engage with you by making eye contact or spend most of the time looking at papers or a computer screen?

If you haven't had a good medical check in a while, make an appointment with your doctor and ask them to check all the basics. Ask for a copy and keep your own records.

- Full blood count
- Electrolytes – kidney and liver function
- Homocysteine – risk of health issues related to methylation
- CRP and ESR – signs of inflammation
- Fasting lipids – LDL & HDL cholesterol and triglycerides
- Fasting blood sugar and insulin
- HBA1c – indication of insulin sensitivity

Establish a good baseline for where you're at now. It helps to prioritise what needs attention and you've got something to measure your progress against. When you're living day to day, things can seem like they're not changing. Once you've recorded where you started, you will be able to look back at any progress and see how far you've come. Beyond that you will start to gain a sense of what works best for you.

If you experience pain give it a number. Rate it out of ten, with one being hardly any and ten being the worst you've ever experienced. Then revisit in a couple of months once you have made some changes. The aim is to re-evaluate, without too much focus on it.

I mentioned it before for measuring sleep but wearing a Fitbit can measure more. It can show improvements in real time: from how far you can walk in a day to measurements of overall fitness. It's really hard to be objective in the moment, but looking back over your progress is helpful to keep you motivated.

Keep a journal if that works best for you. Starting to see results can help you when you can see you are sleeping better, or you're feeling better. Be realistic: a lot of small changes over time will help to understand what works. If you do everything at once not only could it make you worse but you will never know what to blame.

You're an individual. It doesn't matter what other people have or have not been able to do. They're not you. They don't have your individual physiology. They don't have your mindset. They don't have your experience. They don't have your drive or your determination. That's yours and yours alone. And as you develop new insights, act on them like, oh, I realised that when I eat this thing, this happens and maybe this thing is not so good for me. So perhaps I'll find a substitute for that. Be realistic.

- Remove what is harmful
- Swap anything you can't do without to something better
- Optimise sleep and nutrition
- Add in beneficial exercise
- Spend time with other people
- Reduce stress
- Focus on what you want
- Have fun

You can't expect things to change overnight. Remember, it probably took a long time for things to go wrong in order for disease to manifest. It's also going to take some time to reverse-engineer it. Do what it takes so that you can function at your optimal level, wherever that is right now. What is your new normal going to be? You don't know yet, but remain optimistic, be curious. Stay open to what possibilities might be there for you because none of us know what tomorrow will bring. That's a fact.

And remember, whatever you focus on gets bigger. So, focus on what you can achieve, what you can do. And you'll find that that list grows. Let go of anything that doesn't serve you in your journey to be your best self. If you've got people in your life that don't believe that you can do it, you don't have to listen. It's only their opinion, and it may not even be relevant. You matter and self-care is not selfish.

Obviously, your family matters, but if they're not being supportive you can choose to set boundaries. Don't enter into conversations that are not useful and not helpful. You can be assertive without being aggressive. If somebody is not acting in your best interests, you can just nicely say, 'Thank you for sharing that.' Or, 'Thank you, I appreciate that you're only trying to help me, this is my journey.' Practice it to yourself if you need to, and then you'll be able to express yourself better if the time comes.

And remember, overwhelm keeps us stuck. If you're feeling overwhelmed, stop and take a deep breath. Go for a walk and take some time to reset. Trying to do it all at once is almost guaranteed to sabotage your efforts. I would recommend something simple, like adding extra water into your day. Work on improving your sleep, if that's an issue for you. Small steps and consistency add up to big changes over time. Make a decision and be specific. Remember your mind likes detail and will work with you when tell it what you want.

Reread chapters if you have to. Knowledge is power. The mind likes repetition too and it will help to cement your understanding. Remember neurons that fire together, wire together. A little bit like when you're watching a movie again and you might notice something that you didn't see before.

This is all about feeling empowered to make some changes and reap the benefits. Life is for living. Envision your future. What is it that you will do with your new found health and vitality? Where will you be next month, year, decade? Let's see, don't let life pass you by.

Afterword

Good on you for sticking with it and reading to the end. I am impressed! You are definitely in the minority, as many would have given up. It's a lot of information and I'm sure you are an action taker. It's too much to remember from just one reading. That is why I would suggest working through the chapters in order first. Then go back and reread the chapters that stood out at first. Start with the easy changes first, and implement them piece by piece.

If you are travelling this path solo, I wish you every success in your healing. I would love to get an email and hear about how you followed the process. I love supporting you on your path to living the life you deserve.

If you want to find out more about my other offerings keep reading. Download the extras I have for you and check out my website vickirobinson.com.au.

Yours in health,

Vicki xx

About the Author

Vicki Robinson was born in Adelaide, Australia. Her family moved around, following her father's career, before finally settling in Canberra. She is the eldest of four girls who became a pseudo parent to her younger sisters following the untimely death of her father when she was just 14. As a young child, he had always encouraged her to ask questions and explore, to find her own answers. It became a habit that would serve her well throughout her life.

She lives on the beautiful Central Coast of NSW where she enjoys the fresh air and relaxed lifestyle. She values taking time out to enjoy walks on the beach and in the beautiful surrounding bush. Being a keen gardener, she enjoys creating a habitat for local birds, even though they don't always respect her desire to sleep in past 6 am.

Vicki holds Certificates in Nursing – Registered Nurse, Certificate III in Fitness – Aqua and Group Exercise, Certificate IV in Fitness – Personal Trainer, and is a Certified Life & Success Coach, Results Coach, Nutrition and Bio Individual Nutrition Coach, Hypnotherapist – C.Ht, Advanced RTT® Practitioner , Hypnofit® Therapist.

She had always intended to continue with nursing and build on it to provide education on the impact that stress and lifestyle have on our well-being. It's funny how life happens. Sometimes it becomes more about the journey than the destination. Marriage, becoming a new mother and having to face her own health issues set her on a different path.

Becoming a hypnotherapist was not something that she ever planned to do. The sudden end to a 30-year marriage opened up unhealed wounds from her past. Throughout the learning process she healed her past trauma and experienced unexpected improvements in her own health. It led her to the most effective methods to help her clients overcome the blocks that prevented their healing.

Vicki uses the many tools she has acquired, throughout her career, to guide her clients through her 5 Steps to Empowered Self Care program. She believes in education through experience and loves helping individuals to join their own dots. Finding the right solutions and learning to intuitively listen to your body is imperative when it comes to achieving and maintaining good health.

Vicki also provides hypnotherapy to help with specific problems including, but not limited to, pain management, anxiety, lack of motivation and self esteem.

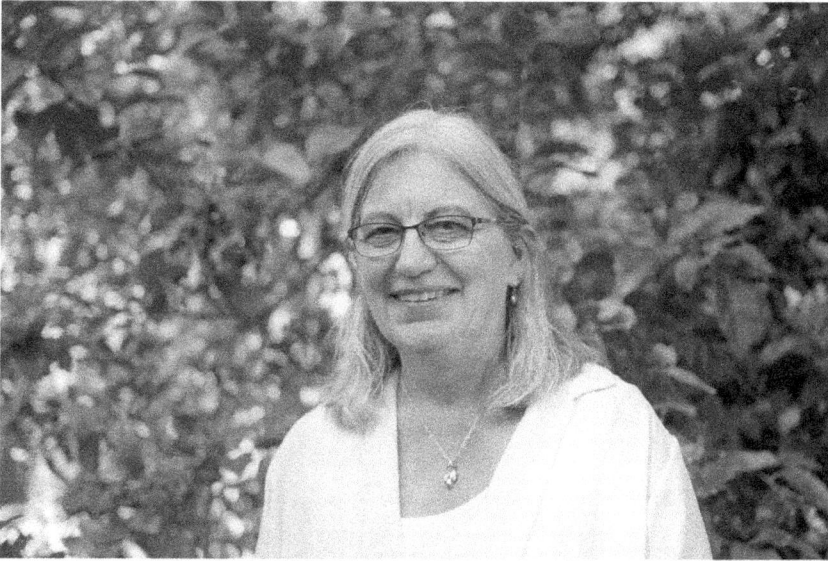

Vicki's website:
www.vickirobinson.com.au
Email: vicki@vickirobinson.com.au

Free Bonus

As promised, I have an Mp3 download for you to listen to. The aim is to give you something to focus on while guiding you through a relaxation. Learning to 'shut off' can be hard. Listening everyday will help to retrain you to relax. Doing so for at least three weeks will help to reinforce the ability. If sleep is an issue it can help with this too. Please be sure that you are in a safe place and do not use while driving or undertaking any activities that require your full attention.

As an extra bonus I also have a food journal that you can download. Keeping track of signs and symptoms is useful when trying to determine if you have any issues related to foods.

You can find your downloads here: vickirobinson.com.au/freebies/

FOOD/MOOD

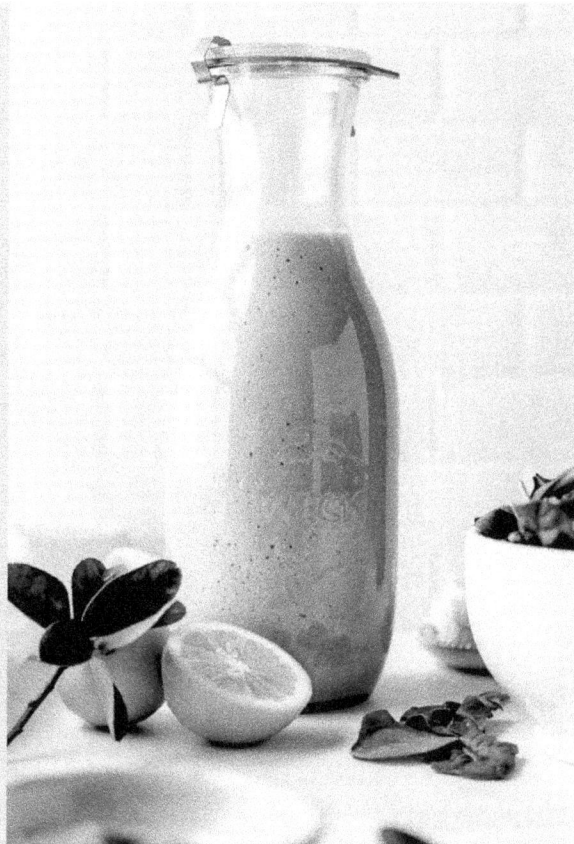

FOOD / MOOD JOURNAL

Vicki Robinson/Holistic Wellness

www.vickirobinson.com.au

VICKI ROBINSON

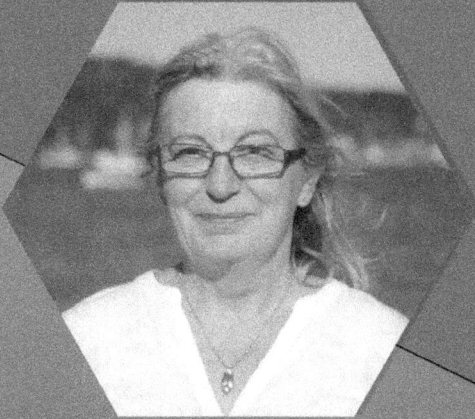

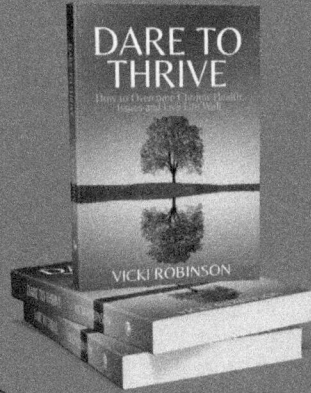

Vicki Robinson, the author of "Dare to Thrive," is a Holistic Wellness Coach and Hypnotherapist. Her passion is empowering people to actively take charge of their health in order to live well. Vicki is well-versed in a broad range of topics related to health and wellness and is an accomplished presenter that easily engages the audience from the get-go.

As a registered nurse and personal trainer, and through her own personal experience of disease, Vicki learned that in order to heal, one needs to take a holistic approach to identify and reverse underlying problems. Vicki leaves her audiences understanding that true health comes through the alignment of personal, emotional, and physical needs.

Vicki has over twenty years' worth of experience in health and fitness. Holding certificates in Nursing, Fitness, Life and Success Coaching, Hypnotherapy and Bio Individual Nutrition her professional grounding paired with her personal experience offers a unique perspective on a range of topics.

Vicki's 3 most popular presentations include Dare to Thrive, Breaking the Stress Cycle and Reverse Metabolic Syndrome, but she can cater a custom presentation for your audience.

DARE TO THRIVE

- Understand the five pillars of health
- Reverse engineer your pillars
- Join the dots to live life well

BREAKING THE STRESS CYCLE

- Understanding where stress comes from
- Key strategies to minimise and eliminate stress
- Remain bulletproof and live stress-free for life

REVERSE METABOLIC SYNDROME

- Understand the mechanics of metabolism
- Three key elements to bring back balance
- Maintain your results for life

To enquire or engage Vicki to speak at your next event, contact details are below

📞 0418 693 026

@ vicki@vickirobinson.com.au

🌐 www.vickirobinson.com.au

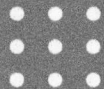

LIVE TO THRIVE Packages

	INDIVIDUAL	GROUP
5 Steps to Empowered Self Care		
Eight week program: Evaluate, Mindset and Stress management, Trauma and resilience, Sleep, Diet and Exercise/Fun, Join the Dots, Live well	✓	✓
Weekly coaching and mentoring calls	✓	✓
Email support	✓	✓
Handouts, checklists	✓	✓
Metabolic Reset		
Twelve week program: Beat sugar/carb cravings, weight management, reverse insulin resistance	✓	✓
Weekly coaching calls	✓	✓
Email support	✓	✓
Handouts, checklists	✓	✓
Bio Individual Nutrition Coaching		
Comprehensive questionnaire and assessment	✓	
Handouts, specific diet guidelines	✓	
Coaching and mentoring calls as required	✓	
Hypnotherapy		
Packages designed to meet individual requirements: Ideal for resistant problems, pain management, stress and trauma. Email and SMS support. Bespoke recording to enhance results	✓	

Vicki Robinson

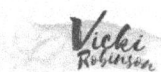

Please contact me at vicki@vickirobinson.com.au with any questions about my services

Thank you for your business!

Notes

www.ingramcontent.com/pod-product-compliance
Lightning Source LLC
Chambersburg PA
CBHW022059020426

42335CB00012B/747